Imaging in Clinical Neurosciences for Non-radiologists

Imaging in Clinical Neurosciences for Non-radiologists

An Atlas

Hemanshu Prabhakar
Professor, Department of Neuroanaesthesiology and Critical Care
All India Institute of Medical Sciences (AIIMS), New Delhi, India

S. Leve Joseph Devarajan
Additional Professor, Department of Neuroimaging & Interventional Neuroradiology
All India Institute of Medical Sciences (AIIMS), New Delhi, India

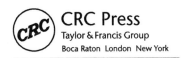

CRC Press
Taylor & Francis Group
Boca Raton London New York

CRC Press is an imprint of the
Taylor & Francis Group, an **informa** business

CRC Press
Boca Raton and London
First edition published 2021
by CRC Press
6000 Broken Sound Parkway NW, Suite 300, Boca Raton, FL 33487-2742

and by CRC Press
2 Park Square, Milton Park, Abingdon, Oxon, OX14 4RN

© 2021 Taylor & Francis Group, LLC
CRC Press is an imprint of Taylor & Francis Group, LLC

Library of Congress Cataloging-in-Publication Data

Names: Prabhakar, Hemanshu, author. | Devarajan, S. Leve Joseph, author.
Title: Imaging in clinical neurosciences for non-radiologists : an atlas / by Hemanshu Prabhakar, S. Leve Joseph Devarajan.
Description: First edition. | Boca Raton, FL : CRC Press, 2021. | Includes index. | Summary: "This Atlas presents both normal and pathological conditions of the Brain and Spine pictorially. Targeted towards non-radiologists, it is a unique book with well labeled and self-explanatory images. All routine conditions involving neuroradiology have been included. Images from different radiological modalities such as X-ray, Computed Tomography (CT), Magnetic Resonance Imaging (MRI) and Digital Subtraction Angiography (DSA) have also been included. This book aims to serve as a ready reckoner for clinicians, trainees, residents as well as professional radiologists"-- Provided by publisher.
Identifiers: LCCN 2020052689 (print) | LCCN 2020052690 (ebook) | ISBN 9780367133306 (hardback) | ISBN 9780367685898 (paperback) | ISBN 9780429025945 (ebook)
Subjects: MESH: Brain Diseases--diagnostic imaging | Spinal Diseases--diagnostic imaging | Brain--anatomy & histology | Spine--anatomy & histology | Atlas
Classification: LCC RC348 (print) | LCC RC348 (ebook) | NLM WL 17 | DDC 616.8/0475--dc23
LC record available at https://lccn.loc.gov/2020052689
LC ebook record available at https://lccn.loc.gov/2020052690

ISBN: 9780367133306 (hbk)
ISBN: 9780367685898 (pbk)
ISBN: 9780429025945 (ebk)

Typeset in Minion Pro
by KnowledgeWorks Global Ltd.

To my family, my teachers and all my students

Hemanshu Prabhakar

To my wife Silviya, kids Bernice & Raphael and my parents

S. Leve Joseph Devarajan

Contents

Preface

A great way of learning is through pictures and images. In medical practice, too, radiology is an extremely important specialty and an essential component in making diagnosis of diseases and various conditions. Neuroradiology unfolds the intricacies of neural structures and, at times, these can be difficult to understand or remember by non-radiologists. The purpose of this book is to collect all possible images of varied neurological problems. Images from different radiological modalities such as x-ray, computed tomography (CT), magnetic resonance imaging (MRI) and digital subtraction angiography (DSA) are included.

The content is entirely pictorial and non-textual. We have tried to ensure each image is well labeled and self-explanatory.

This book covers all common conditions of the brain and spine, both normal and pathological. This book is structured like an atlas, enabling readers to easily understand the various neuroradiological modalities of investigation. Different parts of the normal brain and spine and also the pathologies are presented pictorially with real scans and real cases.

This book should prove useful for trainees, fellows and practitioners related to fields such as neuroanesthesia, neurocritical care, neuroradiology, neurosurgery, and neurology.

Hemanshu Prabhakar
S. Leve Joseph Devarajan

Acknowledgments

We wish to acknowledge the support of the administration of the All India Institute of Medical Sciences (AIIMS), New Delhi, in allowing us to conduct this academic task.

We also thank the faculty and staff of the department of Neuroanaesthesiology and Critical Care and Department of Neuroimaging and Interventional Neuroradiology at AIIMS, for their support.

Special thanks are due to the production team at Taylor & Francis Group, CRC Press: Shivangi, Mouli, Himani, Ritesh, Rajani, Sunaina and Ashraf.

Hemanshu Prabhakar
S. Leve Joseph Devarajan

Authors

Dr. Hemanshu Prabhakar is a Professor in Neuroanaesthesiology and Critical Care at the All India Institute of Medical Sciences (AIIMS), New Delhi, India. He received his training in neuroanaesthesia and completed his PhD at the same institute. He is recipient of the AIIMS Excellence Award 2012 for notable contribution in academics. He has more than 250 publications in national and international journals to his credit. He is a guide and mentor of many DM and PhD students. He is on the Editorial board of *Indian Journal of Palliative care* and is the past Executive Editor of the *Journal of Neuroanaesthesiology and Critical Care*. He is the editor of several books on the subject of neuroanesthesia and neurocritical care. He was featured in the Limca Book of Records 2019.

Dr. S. Leve Joseph Devarajan is an Additional Professor in the Department of Neuroimaging & Interventional Neuroradiology, All India Institute of Medical Sciences (AIIMS), New Delhi, India. He received his training in Neuroimaging and Interventional Neuroradiology from the same institute. He is involved in neurovascular interventional work and is in charge of the in-patient and outpatient services of his department. His special interests include acute stroke intervention, management of pediatric neurovascular diseases, spinal vascular malformations and management of high flow neurovascular malformations. He has around 30 publications to his credit and has contributed chapters to four textbooks. He is a member of various neuroradiology and radiology societies and currently is the Treasurer of Indian Society of Neuroradiology.

List of Abbreviations

NCCT	Non-contrast computed tomography
FLAIR	Fluid-attenuated inversion recovery
CSF	Cerebrospinal fluid
DWI	Diffusion-weighted imaging
FAT SAT	Fat saturation
SWI	Susceptibility weighted imaging
DTI	Diffusion tensor imaging
ADC	Apparent diffusion coefficient
MRS	Magnetic resonance spectroscopy
NMO	Neuromyelitis optica
CBF	Cerebral blood flow
CBV	Cerebral blood volume
MTT	Mean transit time
DSA	Digital subtraction angiography
MCA	Middle cerebral artery
ICA	Internal carotid artery
CVT	Cerebral venous thrombosis
MRV	Magnetic resonance venography
MIP	Maximum intensity projection
TOF MRA	Time of flight magnetic resonance angiography
PA	Postero-anterior
CCA	Common carotid artery
DSC	Dynamic susceptibility contrast
Ax PC	Axial post-contrast
T1 PG	T1 post-gadolinium
ASL	Arterial spin labeling
T1 +C	T1 post contrast
GRE	Gradient-recalled echo
STIR	Short-TI inversion recovery
GCS	Glasgow coma scale
RTA	Road traffic accident
MERGE	Multiple echo recombined gradient echo
LS spine	Lumbo sacral spine
C Spine	Cervical spine

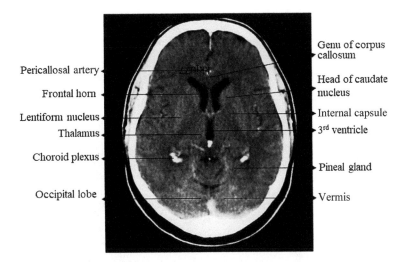

Pericallosal artery

Frontal horn

Lentiform nucleus

Thalamus

Choroid plexus

Occipital lobe

Genu of corpus callosum

Head of caudate nucleus

Internal capsule

3rd ventricle

Pineal gland

Vermis

Figure 1.4 Brain axial section—Lower III ventricular level. Computed tomography scan of brain in axial view at the lower third ventricular level showing normal structures.

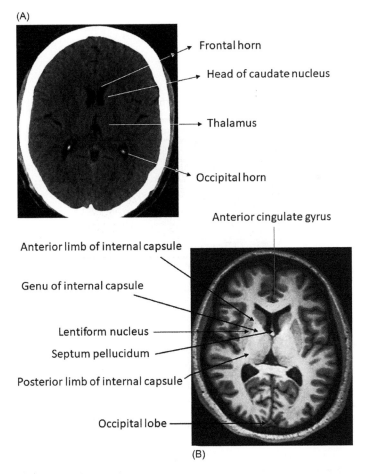

(A)

Frontal horn

Head of caudate nucleus

Thalamus

Occipital horn

Anterior cingulate gyrus

Anterior limb of internal capsule

Genu of internal capsule

Lentiform nucleus

Septum pellucidum

Posterior limb of internal capsule

Occipital lobe

(B)

Figure 1.5 Brain axial section—Upper III ventricular level: **(A)** Computed tomography scan of brain in axial view at the upper third ventricular level showing normal structures. **(B)** Magnetic resonance imaging of brain in axial view at the upper third ventricular level showing normal structures.

(A)

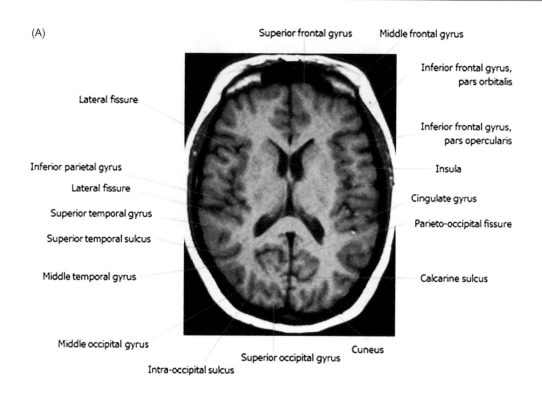

(B)

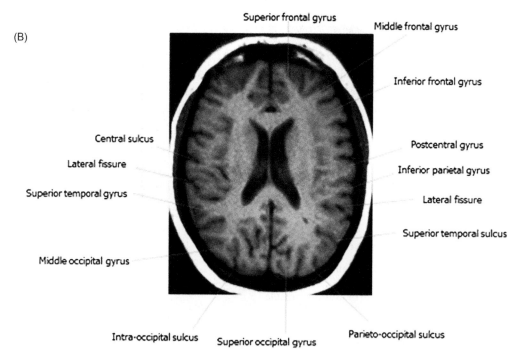

Figure 1.6 Brain axial section—Magnetic resonance imaging of brain in axial view at the upper third ventricular and body of the lateral ventricles levels respectively showing normal structures.

List of Contributors

Dr. Parthiban Balasundaram (Associate Consultant)
Department of Neuroimaging & Interventional Radiology, MGM Healthcare, Chennai, India.

Dr. Manoj Kumar Nayak (Senior Resident)
Department of Neuroimaging & Interventional Neuroradiology, All India Institute of Medical Sciences, New Delhi, India.

Dr. Kalyan Sarma (Senior Resident)
Department of Neuroimaging & Interventional Neuroradiology, All India Institute of Medical Sciences, New Delhi, India

Normal anatomy

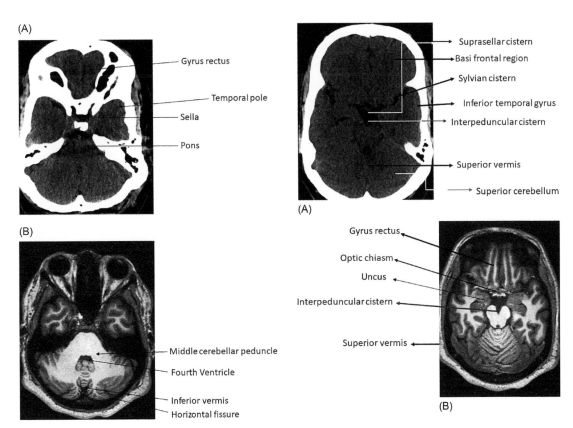

Figure 1.1 Brain axial section—Pons level:
(A) Computed tomography scan of brain in axial view at the level of pons showing normal structures. **(B)** Magnetic resonance imaging of brain in axial view at the level of pons showing normal structures.

Figure 1.2 Brain axial section—Midbrain level:
(A) Computed tomography scan of brain in axial view at the level of midbrain and suprasellar cistern showing normal structures. **(B)** Magnetic resonance imaging of brain in axial view at the same level showing normal structures.

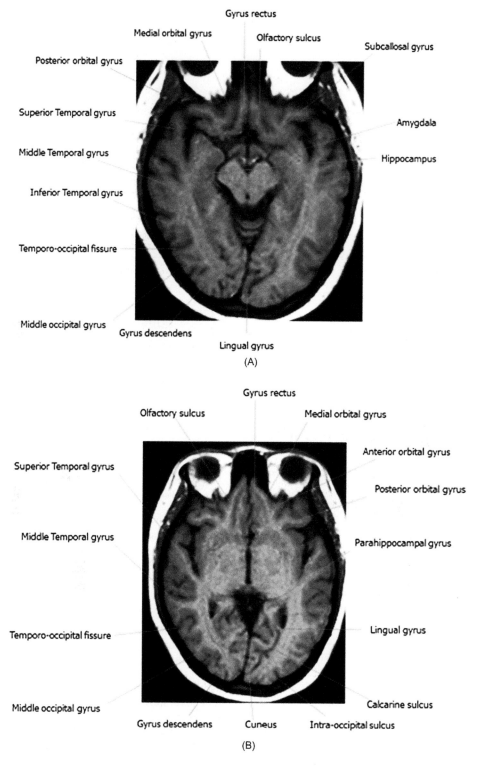

Figure 1.3 Brain axial section—Upper midbrain and lower III ventricle levels: (**A** and **B**) Magnetic resonance imaging of brain in axial view at the upper midbrain and lower third ventricle levels showing normal structures.

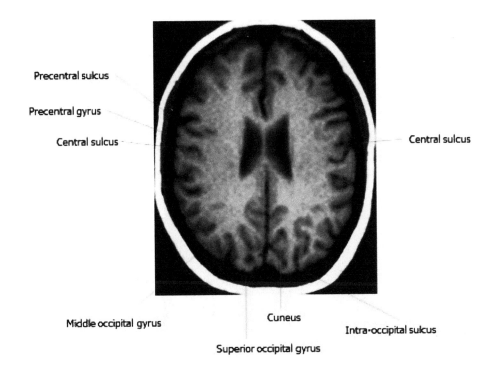

Precentral sulcus

Precentral gyrus

Central sulcus

Central sulcus

Middle occipital gyrus

Cuneus

Intra-occipital sulcus

Superior occipital gyrus

Superior frontal gyrus

Middle frontal gyrus

Inferior frontal gyrus

Superior frontal sulcus

Centrum semiovale

Central sulcus

Central sulcus

Postcentral sulcus

Postcentral sulcus

Supramarginal gyrus

Intraparietal sulcus

Angular gyrus

Parietooccipital sulcus

Superior parietal gyrus

Precuneus

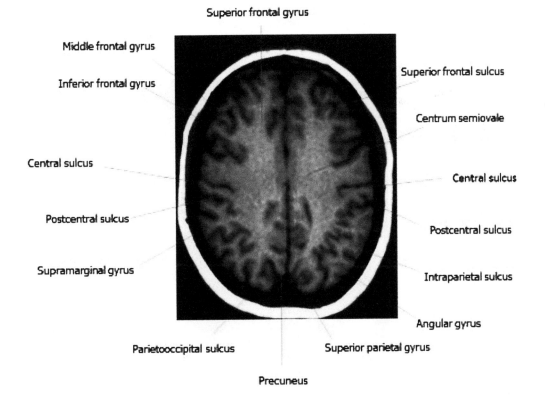

Figure 1.7 Brain axial section—Magnetic resonance imaging of brain in axial view at the centrum semiovale level showing normal structures.

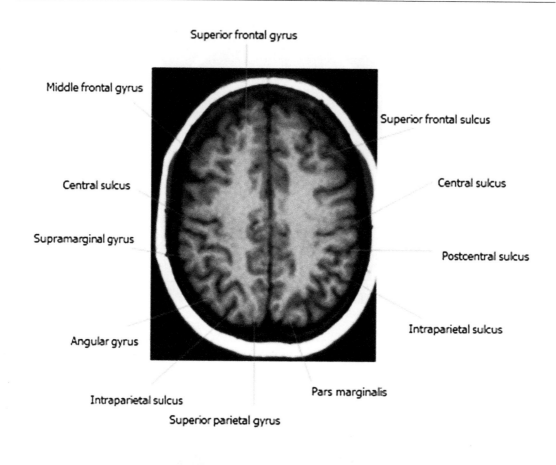

Superior frontal gyrus

Middle frontal gyrus

Superior frontal sulcus

Central sulcus

Central sulcus

Supramarginal gyrus

Postcentral sulcus

Angular gyrus

Intraparietal sulcus

Intraparietal sulcus

Pars marginalis

Superior parietal gyrus

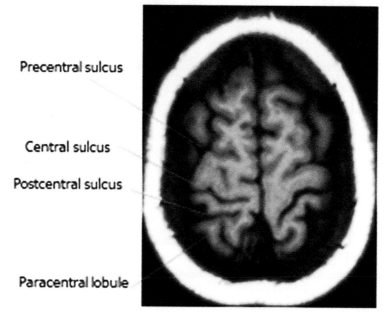

Precentral sulcus

Central sulcus

Postcentral sulcus

Paracentral lobule

Figure 1.8 Brain axial section—High frontoparietal. Magnetic resonance imaging of brain in axial view at the high frontoparietal levels showing normal structures.

(A)

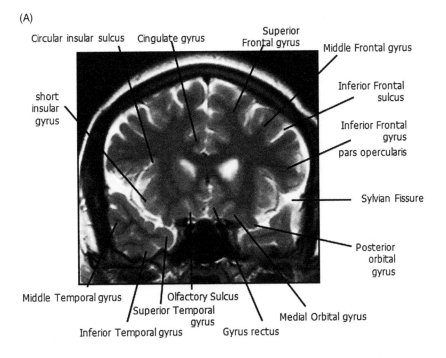

Circular insular sulcus   Cingulate gyrus   Superior Frontal gyrus   Middle Frontal gyrus

short insular gyrus

Inferior Frontal sulcus

Inferior Frontal gyrus pars opercularis

Sylvian Fissure

Posterior orbital gyrus

Middle Temporal gyrus   Olfactory Sulcus   Medial Orbital gyrus
Superior Temporal gyrus
Inferior Temporal gyrus   Gyrus rectus

(B)

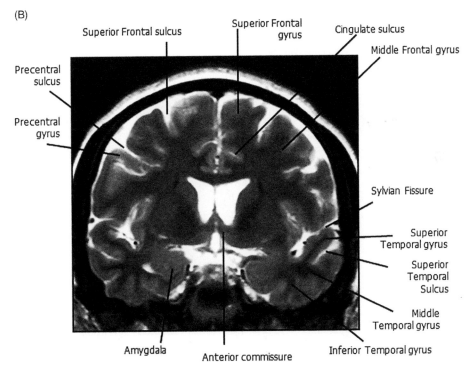

Superior Frontal sulcus   Superior Frontal gyrus   Cingulate sulcus

Middle Frontal gyrus

Precentral sulcus

Precentral gyrus

Sylvian Fissure

Superior Temporal gyrus

Superior Temporal Sulcus

Middle Temporal gyrus

Amygdala   Anterior commissure   Inferior Temporal gyrus

Figure 1.9 Brain coronal section—Frontal lobes level: **(A)** and **(B)** Magnetic resonance imaging of brain in coronal section at the level of frontal horns showing normal structures.

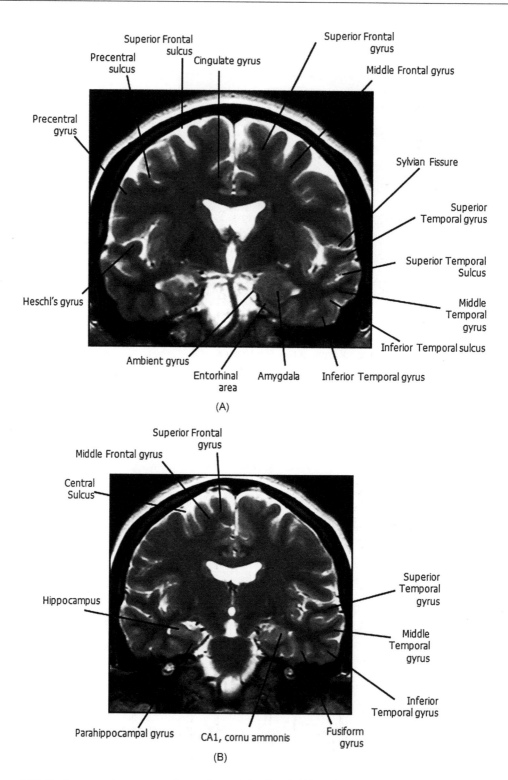

Figure 1.10 Brain coronal sections—Lateral ventricles level: **(A)** and **(B)** Magnetic resonance imaging of brain in coronal section at the level of body of lateral ventricles showing normal structures.

(A)

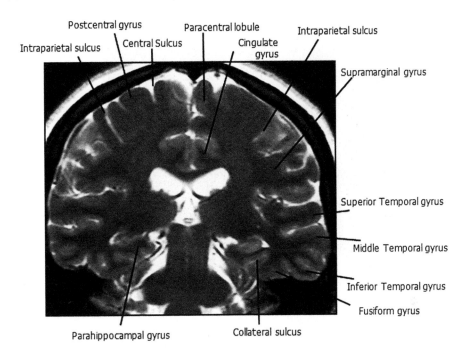

(B)

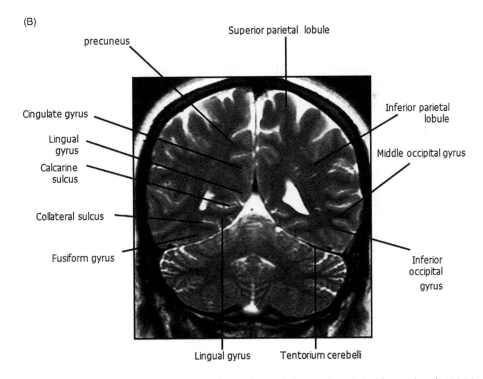

Figure 1.11 Brain coronal sections—Posterior lateral ventricles and occipital horns level: **(A)** Magnetic resonance imaging of brain in coronal section at the level of posterior lateral ventricles showing normal structures. **(B)** Magnetic resonance imaging of brain in coronal section at the level of occipital horns showing normal structures.

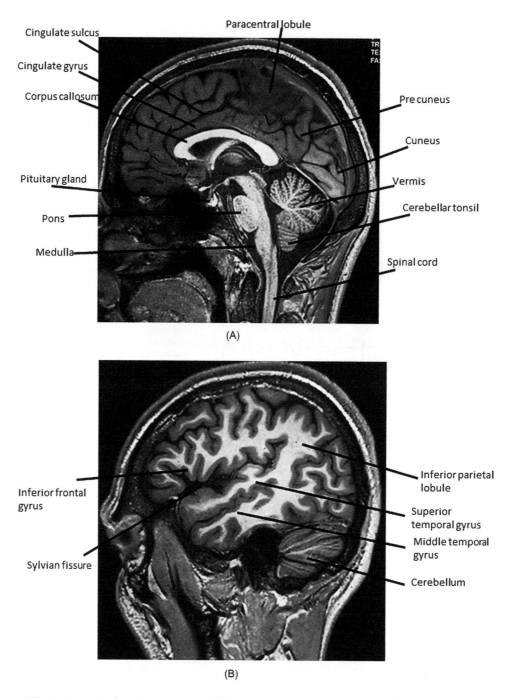

Figure 1.12 Brain sagittal section: **(A)** and **(B)** Magnetic resonance imaging of brain in mid-sagittal and parasagittal sections showing normal structures.

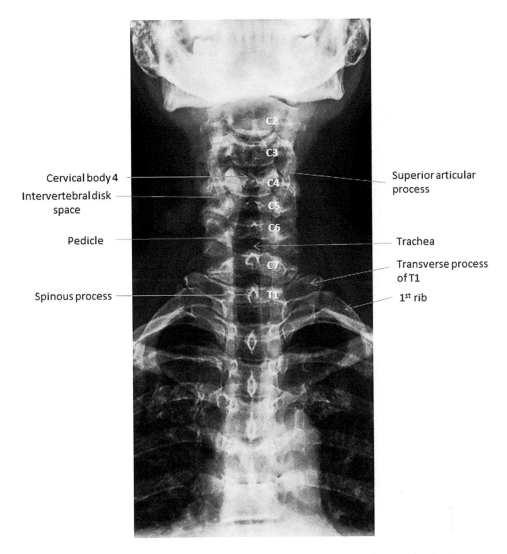

Figure 1.13 Spine X-ray of cervical spine—Anteroposterior view: X-ray of cervical spine in anteroposterior view showing normal vertebral structures.

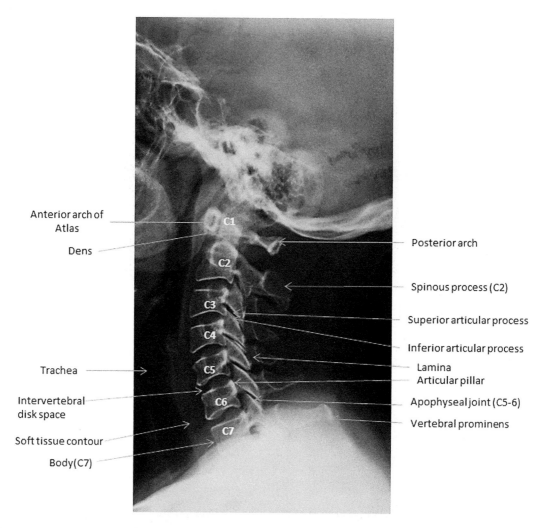

Anterior arch of Atlas

Dens

Posterior arch

Spinous process (C2)

Superior articular process

Inferior articular process

Trachea

Lamina
Articular pillar

Intervertebral disk space

Apophyseal joint (C5-6)

Vertebral prominens

Soft tissue contour

Body (C7)

Figure 1.14 Spine X-ray of cervical spine—Lateral view: X-ray of cervical spine in lateral view showing normal vertebral structures.

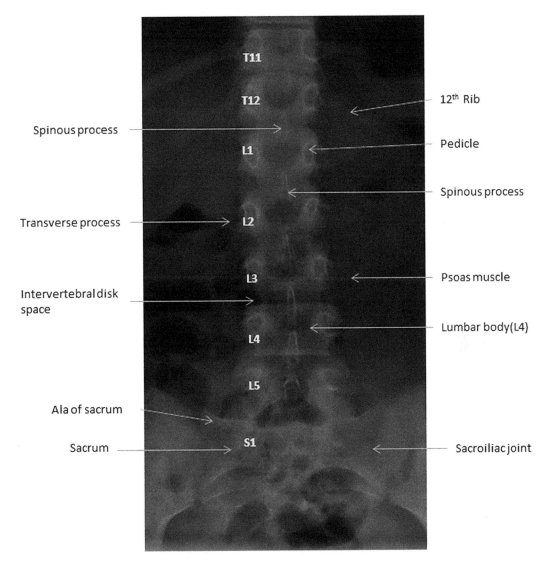

Figure 1.15 Spine X-ray of lumbosacral spine—Anteroposterior view: X-ray of lumbosacral spine in anteroposterior view showing normal vertebral structures.

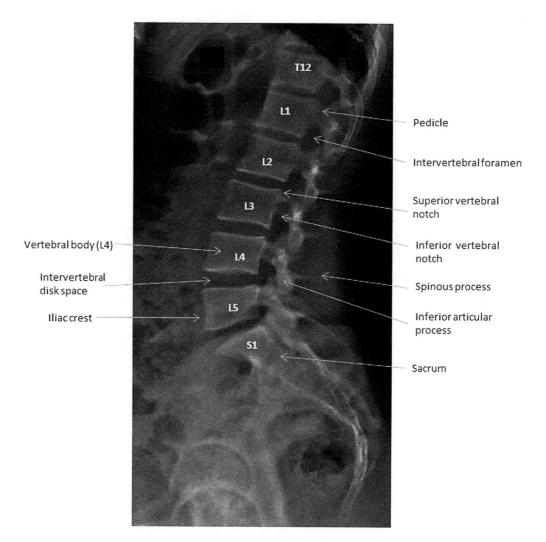

Figure 1.16 Spine X-ray of lumbosacral spine—Lateral view: X-ray of lumbosacral spine in lateral view showing normal vertebral structures.

2

Congenital anomalies

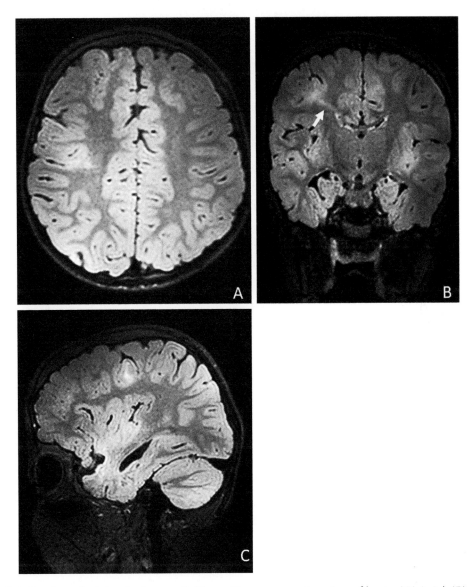

Figure 2.1 Focal cortical dysplasia type 2: Magnetic resonance imaging of brain. **(A)** Axial, **(B)** coronal and **(C)** sagittal FLAIR images showing subcortical and deep white matter hyperintense signal in the depth of the sulcus with adjacent gyral thickening.

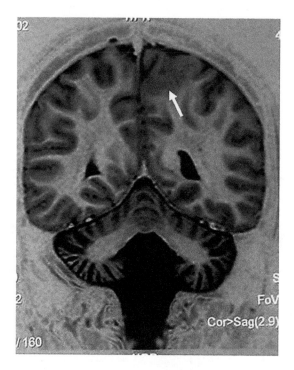

Figure 2.2 Focal cortical dysplasia type 1: Coronal inversion recovery image shows thickening of the left medial parietal cortex with loss of demarcation between grey and white matter without any mass effect.

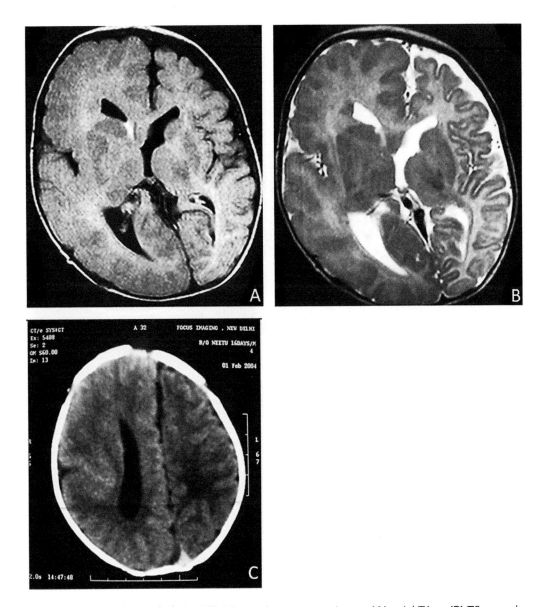

Figure 2.3 Hemimegalencephaly (HME): Magnetic resonance image **(A)** axial T1-w, **(B)** T2-w, and **(C)** non-contrast computed tomography images show dysmorphic enlargement of right cerebral hemisphere with abnormal gyration and shallow sulcation. Note the consequence shifting of falx to left side. Body and occipital horn of right lateral ventricle are also enlarged. Ipsilateral ventricular enlargement is characteristic finding. HME is a disorder of cortical development, more specifically neuroglial proliferation.

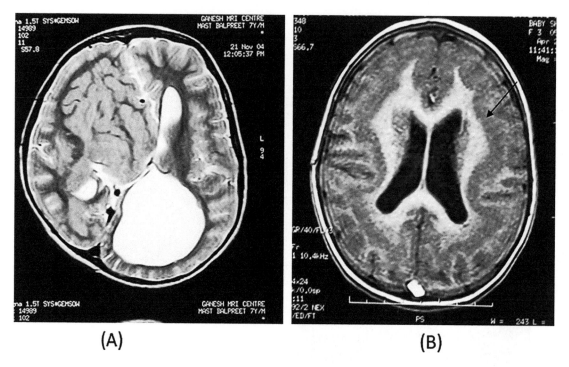

(A)   (B)

Figure 2.4 Subcortical heterotopia: **(A)** Axial T2-w image shows subcortical large focal mass of heterotopic grey matter, thin overlying cortex and deformed underlying ventricle. Paucity of white matter in left parietal lobe and asymmetrical dilatation of body of left lateral ventricle is also seen. **(B)** Axial T1-w image shows bilateral subcortical band (black arrow) of heterotopic grey matter with thin outer cortex. Heterotopias are disorders of abnormal neuronal migration.

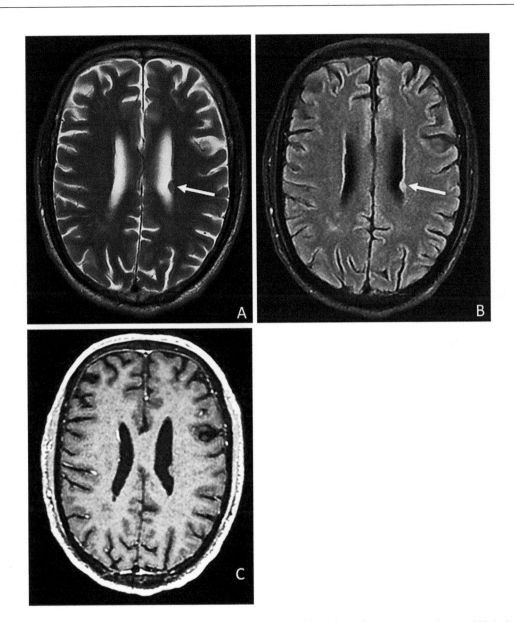

Figure 2.5 Periventricular nodular heterotopia: A 34-year-old male with recurrent seizures. **(A)** Axial T2-w and **(B)** FLAIR images show a small subependymal nodule related to the lateral wall of left lateral ventricle (white arrow). **(C)** Axial T1-w post-gadolinium image show no enhancement. It shows signal similar to normal appearing cortex in all sequences.

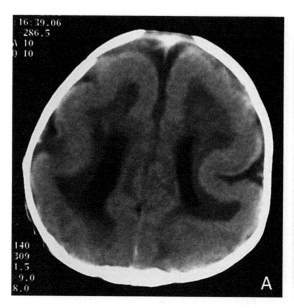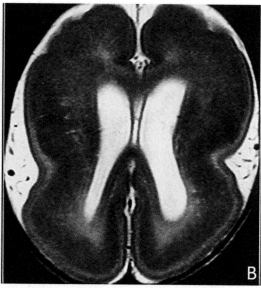

Figure 2.6 Lissencephaly: **(A)** Axial NCCT image shows absence of normal grey-white matter differentiation with diffuse flattening of sulci and single prominent sulcation in the region of Sylvian fissure. Ventricles are slightly dysmorphic in appearance. **(B)** Axial T2-w image shows a figure of 8 appearance of brain parenchyma with near complete lack of sulcation throughout cortex with uniform thickening of cortical grey matter and smooth cortical surface (pachygyria). Diffuse prominence of lateral ventricles is seen. Lissencephaly is the disorder of abnormal neuronal proliferation and migration, and represents a spectrum of disorder which can be associated with microcephaly and band heterotopia.

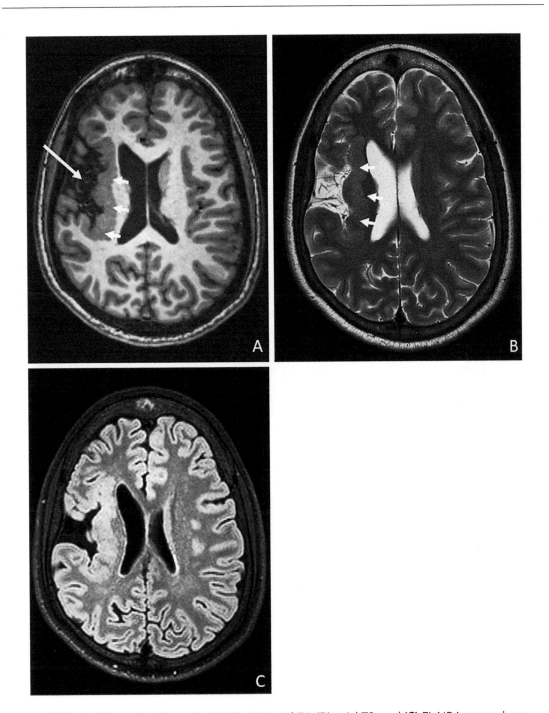

Figure 2.7 Perisylvian polymicrogyria (PMG): **(A)** Axial T1, **(B)** axial T2, and **(C)** FLAIR images show malformed right Sylvian fissure (white long arrow) which is wide open, with cortical thickening. Cortex shows lumpy and bumpy contour (white short arrows). Cortex shows signal similar to the normal appearing cortex elsewhere. PMG represents abnormal cortical development during the late stage of neuronal migration and organization.

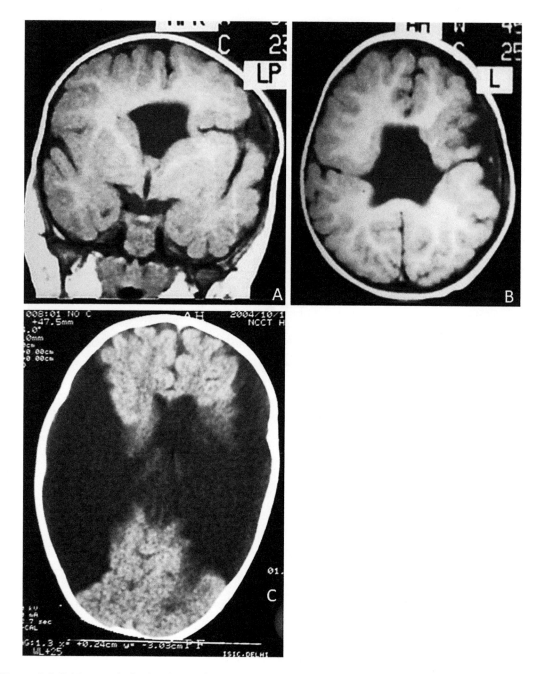

Figure 2.8 Schizencephaly: **(A)** Coronal and **(B)** axial T1-w images show bilateral grey matter-lined cleft in posterior frontal lobes extending from ventricular margin to cortical surface with apposed cleft walls. **(C)** Axial NCCT image shows bilateral grey matter-lined clefts extending from ventricular margin to cortical surface with widely separated and CSF filled cleft walls.

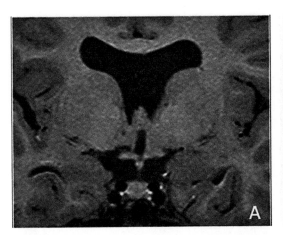 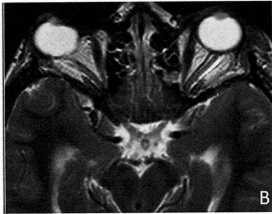

Figure 2.9 Septo-optic dysplasia (SOD): **(A)** Coronal T1-w and **(B)** axial T2-w images show absent septum pellucidum, squared off frontal horns with inferior pointing of the ventricles, hypoplastic pituitary stalk and hypoplastic optic nerves.

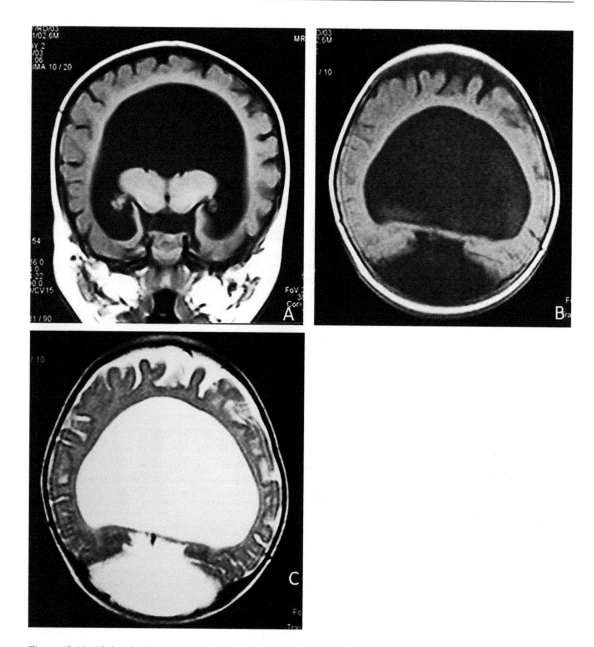

Figure 2.10 Alobar holoprosencephaly: **(A)** Coronal, **(B)** axial T1-w, and **(C)** axial T2-w images show large single midline monoventricle, thin cortical mantle, and fused thalami. Septum pellucidum, third ventricle, interhemispheric fissure and falx cerebri are absent. CSF intensity dorsal cyst is also seen. Holoprosencephaly represents anomaly in midline cleavage and differentiation of ventral prosencephalon. Alobar is the most severe form.

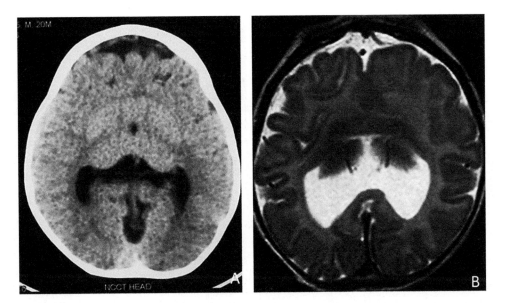

Figure 2.11 Semilobar holoprosencephaly: **(A)** Axial NCCT and **(B)** axial T2-w images show fused lateral ventricles with absence of septum pellucidum, partially developed occipital horns and third ventricle and partially fused thalami. Incompletely formed interhemispheric fissure is seen with absent falx cerebri anteriorly.

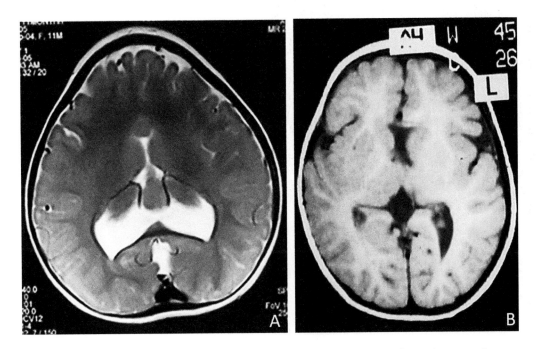

Figure 2.12 Lobar holoprosencephaly: **(A)** Axial T2-w and **(B)** T1-w images show absence of septum pellucidum with fusion of frontal horns of bilateral lateral ventricles communicating with third ventricle. Corpus callosum is hypoplastic.

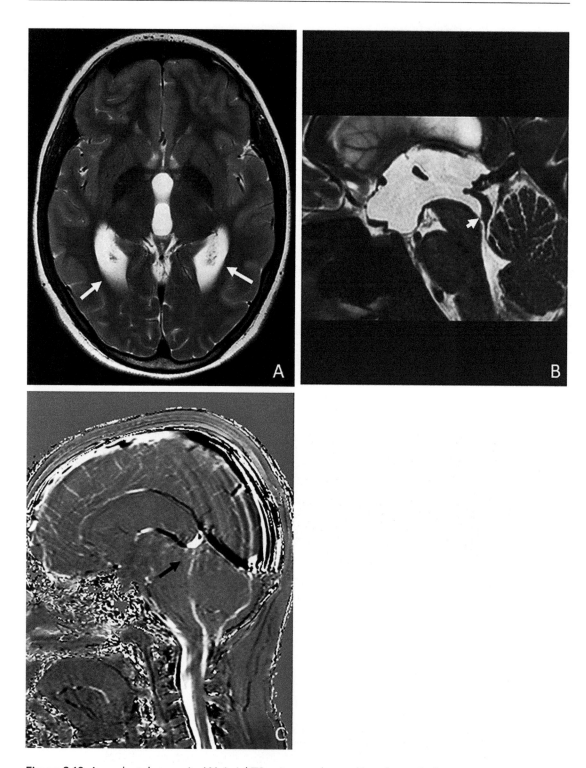

Figure 2.13 Aqueductal stenosis: **(A)** Axial T2-w image shows dilated ventricular system suggestive of hydrocephalus (white long arrows). **(B)** Sagittal DRIVE image shows narrowing of distal aqueduct by a septum (white short arrow). **(C)** Sagittal phase contrast CSF flow study shows no flow across the aqueduct (black arrow). Flowing CSF is seen either as dark and white depending upon the direction of the flow.

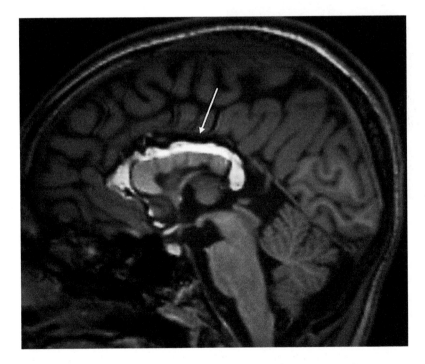

Figure 2.14 Corpus callosal agenesis: **(A)** Axial T1-w and **(B)** sagittal T2-w images show complete absence of corpus callosum, absent cingulate sulcus with medial hemispheric sulci seen reaching third ventricle in a radial fashion, with dilated high riding third ventricle and parallel configuration of lateral ventricles (colpocephaly indicated by black arrow).

Figure 2.15 Corpus callosal lipoma: Sagittal T1-w image shows hyperintense linear mass overlying the corpus callosum (white arrow).

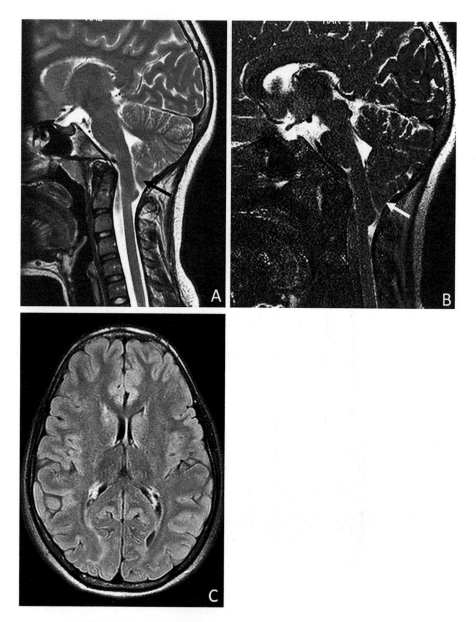

Figure 2.16 Arnold-Chiari malformation type I: **(A)** Sagittal T2-w image shows inferior displacement of peg-shaped tonsils beyond the level of foramen magnum (black arrow). **(B)** Sagittal DRIVE image shows effacement of CSF space at the level of posterior foramen magnum (white arrow). **(C)** Axial FLAIR image shows no hydrocephalus in this case, though it is a common association with ACM.

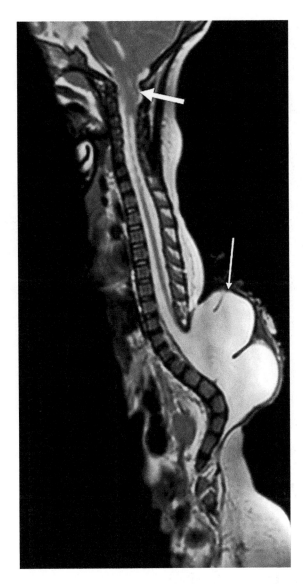

Figure 2.17 Arnold-Chiari malformation type II: Sag T2 image shows dorsal herniation of meningeal sac and nerve roots suggesting lumbosacral myelomeningocele (thin white arrow) with inferior displacement of tonsils (thick white arrow) beyond the level of foramen magnum.

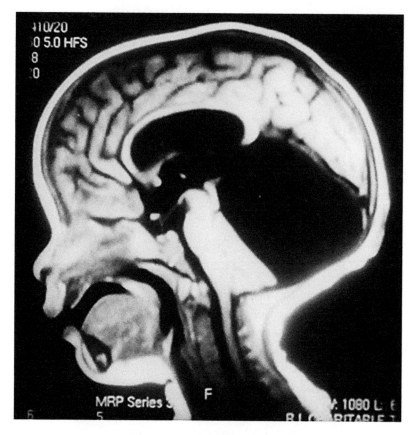

Figure 2.18 Dandy-Walker malformation: Sagittal FLAIR image shows enlarged posterior fossa with large posterior fossa cyst causing compression of vermis and fourth ventricle.

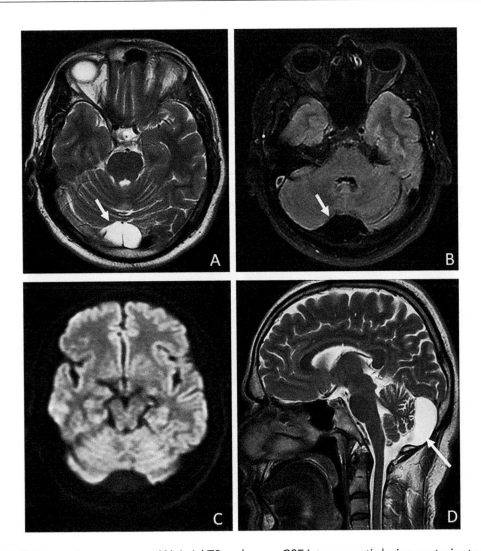

Figure 2.19 Mega cisterna magna: **(A)** Axial T2-w shows a CSF intense cystic lesion posterior to the cerebellum (white arrows). It shows a linear septation within, thus differentiating from arachnoid cyst. **(B)** Axial FLAIR image shows complete suppression of the contents. **(C)** Axial DWI shows hypointense signal similar to CSF, suggestive of diffusion facilitation. **(D)** Sagittal T2-w image shows well-defined CSF intense structure posterior to cerebellum without any mass effect.

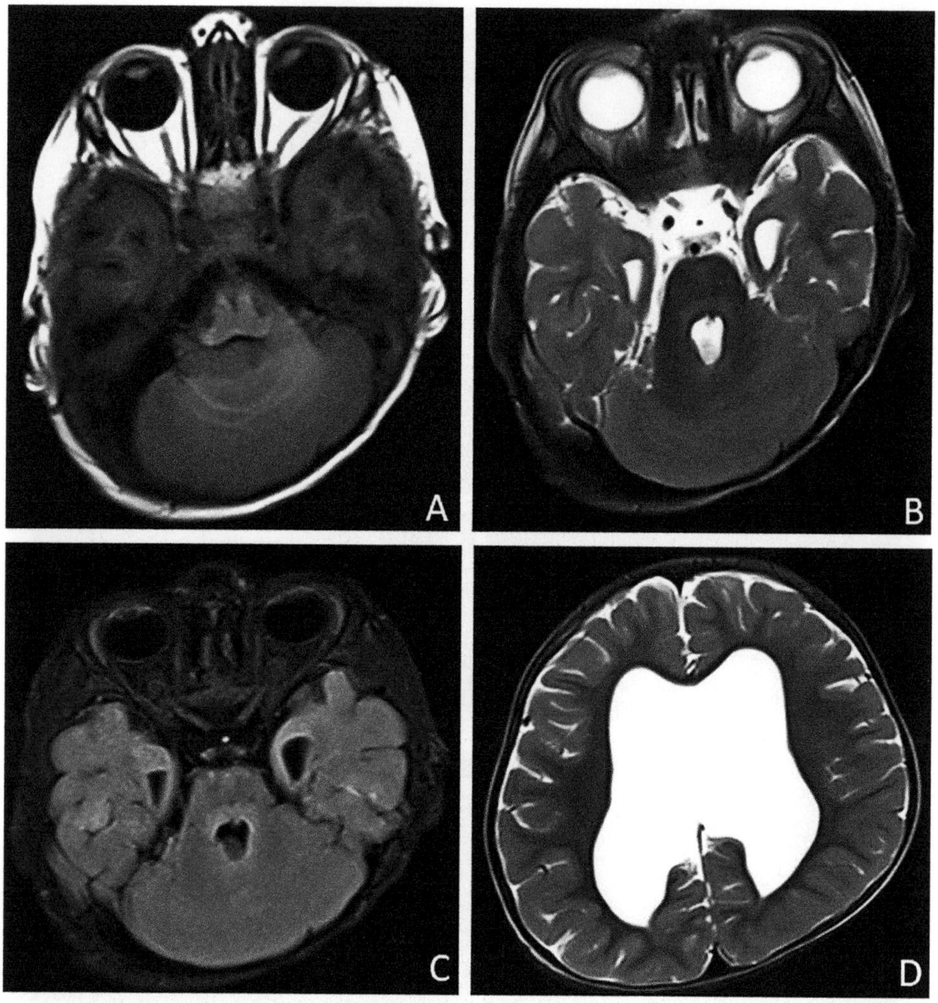

Figure 2.20 Rhombencephalosynapsis: **(A)** Axial T1-w, **(C)** T2-w, and **(B, D)** FLAIR images show absence of vermis with fusion of cerebellar hemispheres with transversely oriented cerebellar folia. Fourth ventricle appears diamond shaped with dilatation of lateral ventricles.

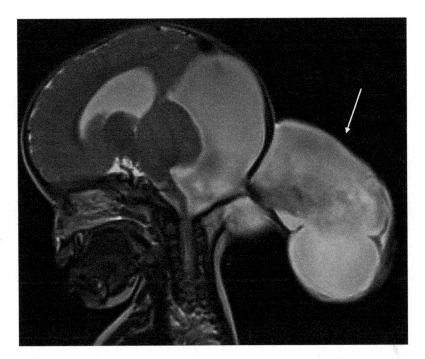

Figure 2.21 Occipital cephalocele: Sagittal T2-w image shows enlarged posterior fossa containing a giant cyst communicating with herniated meninges in the occipital region with elevation of torcular herophili and hypoplastic vermis. Thinning of corpus callosum is also seen.

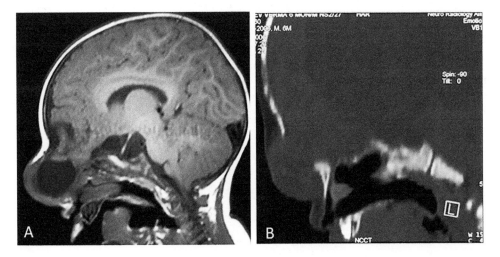

Figure 2.22 Nasoethmoidal and frontal and nasal cephalocele: **(A)** Sagittal T1-w and **(B)** NCCT (bone window) images show herniation of CSF intensity sac along with basifrontal lobe extending through the floor of anterior cranial fossa midline defect just above the nasal bone in the region of foramen cecum. It is seen producing a midline nasal mass.

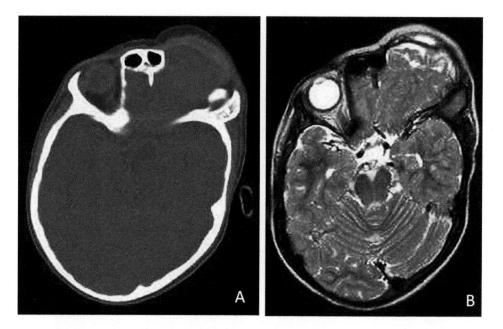

Figure 2.23 Orbital encephalocele: (A) Axial NCCT and (B) T2-w image shows the hypoplastic greater wing of left sphenoid bone with large bone defect and left basifrontal lobe protruding into the left orbit.

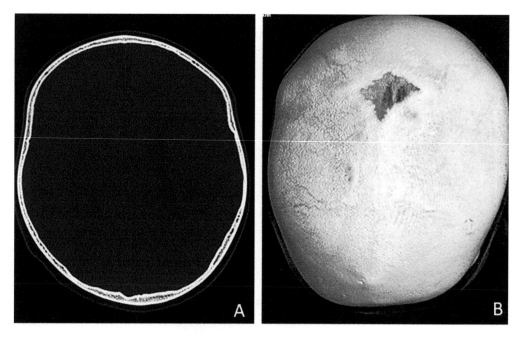

Figure 2.24 Craniosynostosis: **(A)** Axial NCCT (bone window) and **(B)** 3D volume-rendered images show fusion of sagittal, coronal, and lambdoid sutures.

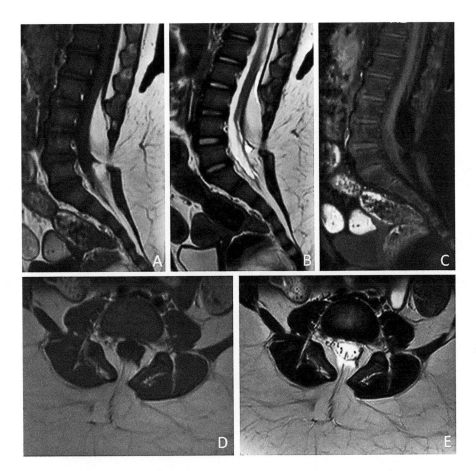

Figure 2.25 Lipomyelocele with LLTC: **(A)** Sagittal T1-w and **(B)** T2-w images show posterior bony defect through which subcutaneous fat is entering the spinal canal. **(C)** Cord is low lying and tethered to the fatty mass. **(D)** Axial T1-w and **(E)** T2-w images show lower lumbar posterior bony defect and fatty mass.

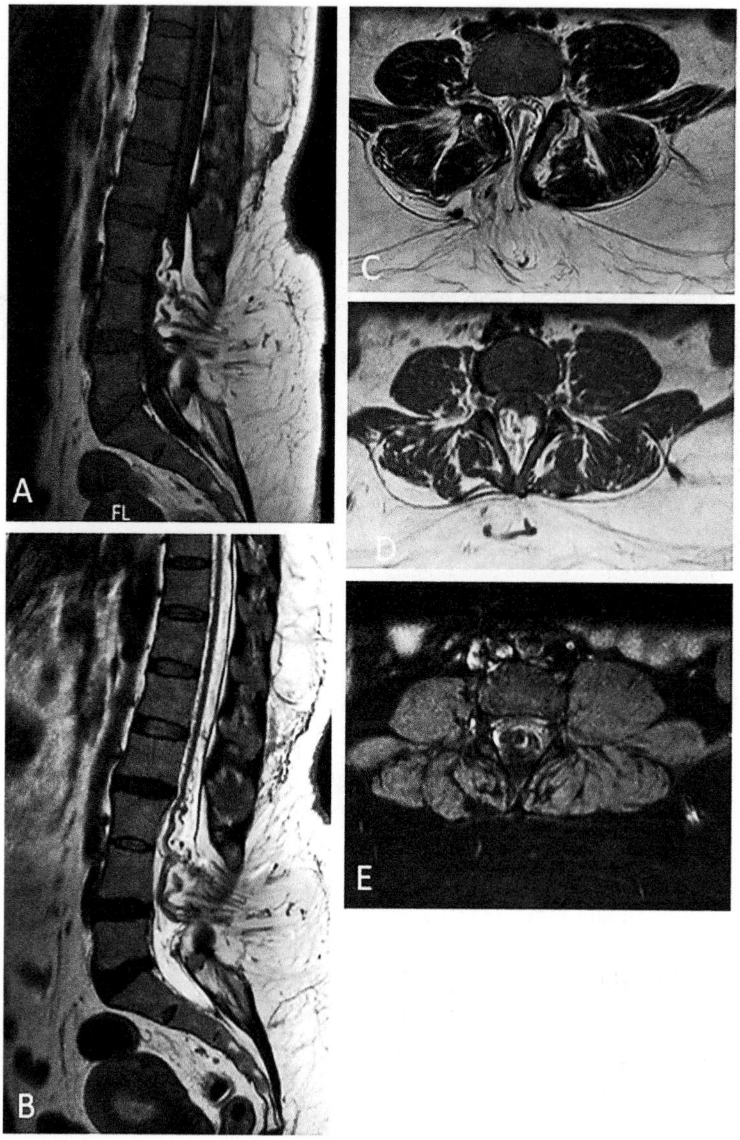

Figure 2.26 Lipomyelocele with arteriovenous malformation (AVM): **(A)** Sagittal T1 & **(B)** saggital T2, **(C)** axial T1-w, **(D)** axial T2-w and **(E)** axial T1 fat saturated images show large posterior bony defect, with low lying cord tethered to the fat. Multiple flow voids are seen both within and outside the dural sac indicating feeding arteries and draining veins of AVM.

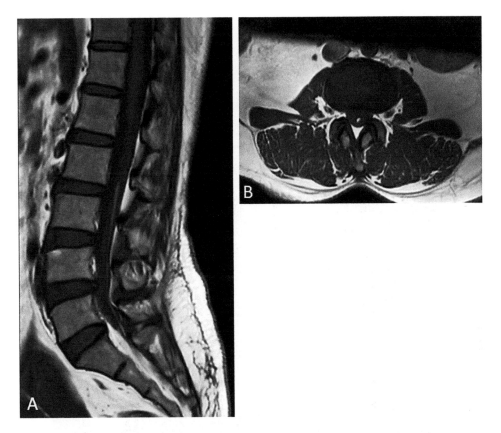

Figure 2.27 Fatty filum terminale: **(A)** Sagittal and **(B)** axial T1-w images show linear hyperintense lesion along the filum terminale. Note the closed dural sac and absent posterior bony defect differentiating it from lipomyelocele.

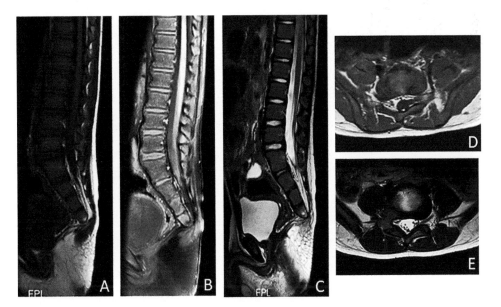

Figure 2.28 Sacral agenesis and filar lipoma: **(A)** Saggital T1, **(B)** saggital FAT SAT, **(C)** saggital T2, **(D)** axial T1, and **(E)** axial T2 images show low-lying tethered cord with lower sacral agenesis. Axial T1-w image shows filum terminal appearing thick and hyperintense.

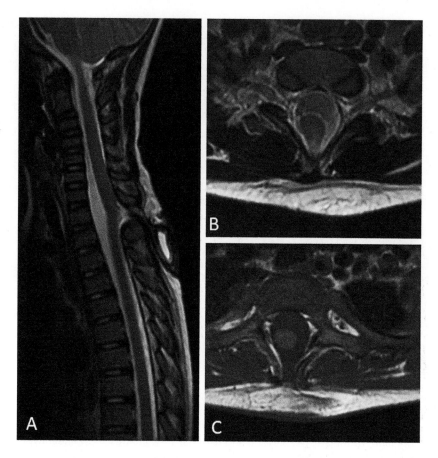

Figure 2.29 Atretic myelocystocele: **(A)** Saggital T2, **(B)** axial T1, and **(C)** axial T2 images show atretic subcutaneous sac with posterior tethering of the cord extending through spina bifida at the level of D1 vertebra.

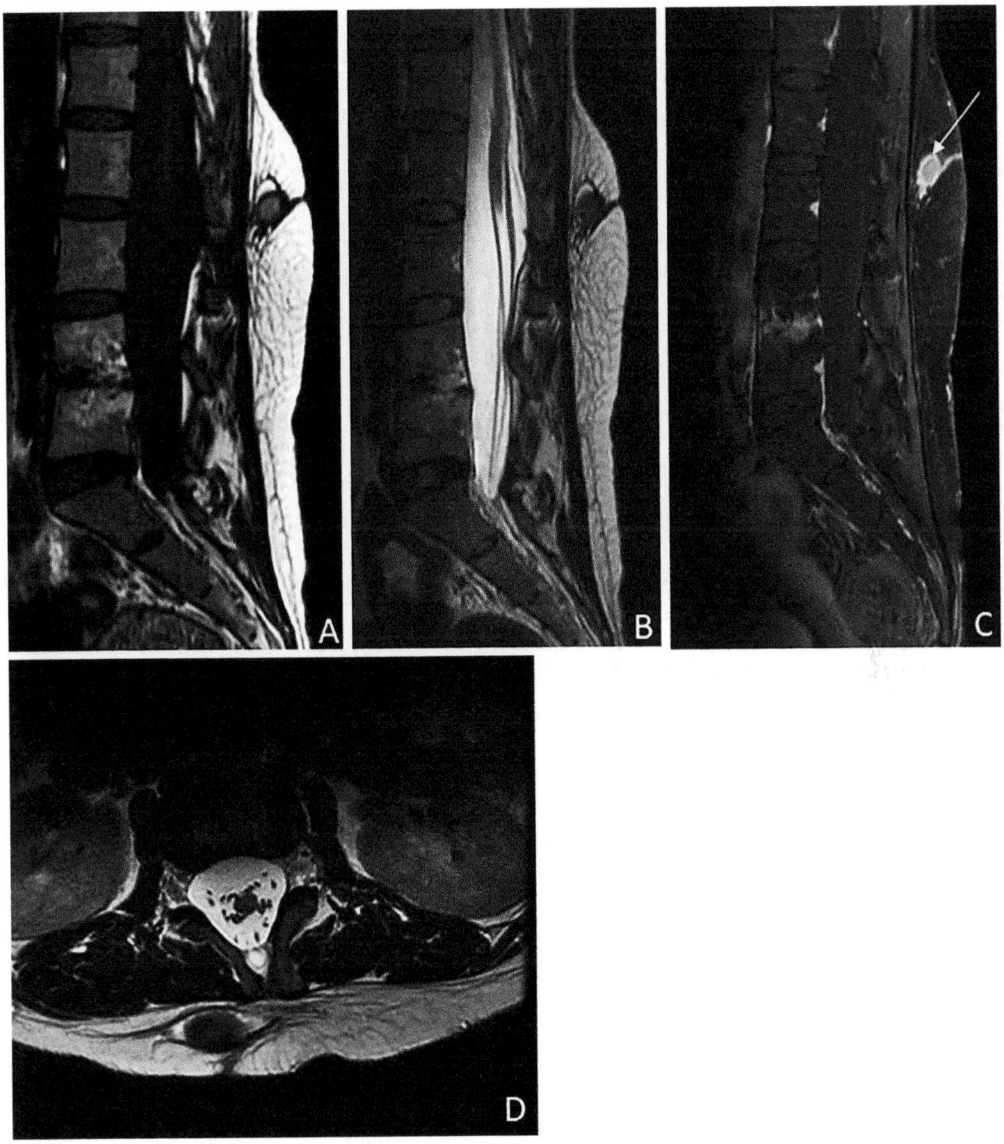

Figure 2.30 Dorsal dermal sinus: **(A)** Saggital T1, **(B)** saggital T2, **(C)** saggital T1+C, and **(D)** axial T2 images shows low-lying tethered cord with dorsal dermal sinus extending posteriorly into intensely enhancing cystic lesion at L2-L3 level, likely infected dermoid cyst(white arrow). There is also evidence of unrelated L4-L5 spondylodiscitis.

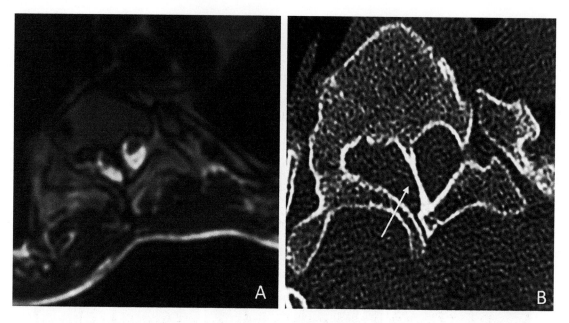

Figure 2.31 Split cord malformation type I: **(A)** Axial T2-w and **(B)** NCCT bone window images show duplicated dural sacs with midline osseous spur (white arrow) and associated spina bifida.

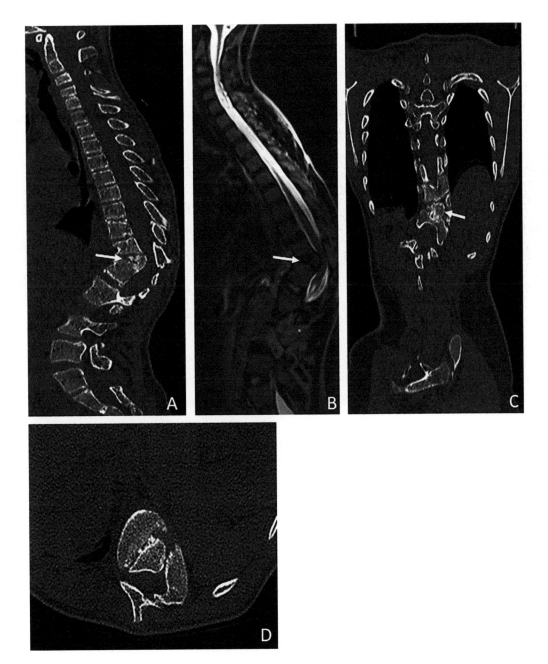

Figure 2.32 Vertebral segmentation anomaly: **(A)** Sagittal NCCT reconstruction of spine, **(B)** sagittal T2 image, and **(C)** coronal NCCT reconstruction of the spine show hemivertebra at D10 level (white arrows) and scoliosis at lower dorsal level with convexity to right side. **(D)** Axial NCCT image shows non-fusion of posterior elements.

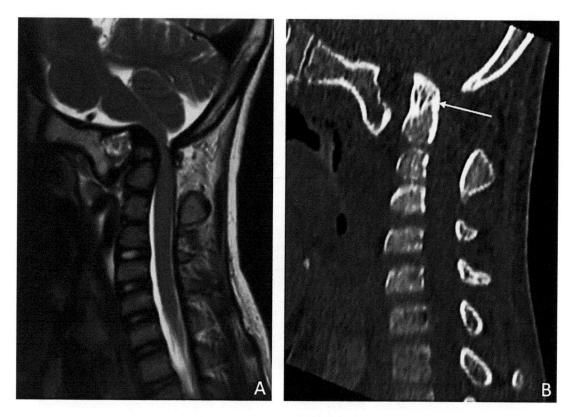

Figure 2.33 Basilar invagination (BI): **(A)** Sagittal T2w and **(B)** NCCT bone window images show tip of dens lying above the level of foramen magnum (white arrow), atlanto-occipital assimilation and atlanto-axial dislocation with increased anterior atlanto-dental interval and decreased posterior atlanto-dental interval causing foramen magnum stenosis with effacement of perimedullary CSF spaces and compression of cervicomedullary junction.

3

Epilepsy imaging

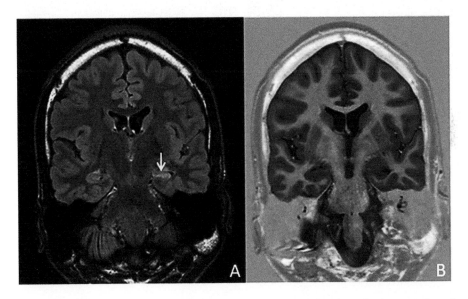

Figure 3.1 Mesial temporal sclerosis: A 32-year-old man presented with multiple episodes of complex partial seizures for 8 years. **(A)** Coronal FLAIR images show bright signal involving left hippocampus which shows volume loss as better seen in **(B)** T1 inversion recovery (IR) image. These features are classical of Hippocampal or medial temporal sclerosis which is a common cause of surgically treatable refractory epilepsy.

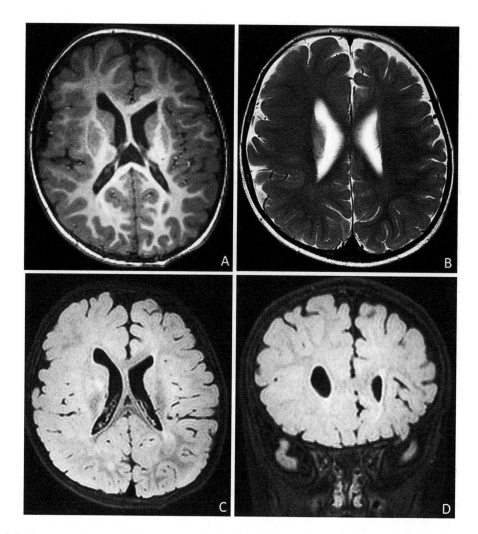

Figure 3.2 Hemimegalencephaly: A 3-year-old male presented with multiple episodes of seizures since birth. **(A)** Axial T1, **(B)** T2, and **(C)** FLAIR images show hypertrophy of right anterior temporal, frontal lobe, insula and basal ganglia with T2/FLAIR hyperintense signal in adjacent white matter. **(D)** Coronal FLAIR image shows enlarged right frontal lobe with white matter signal changes. Note is made of enlargement of right lateral ventricle.

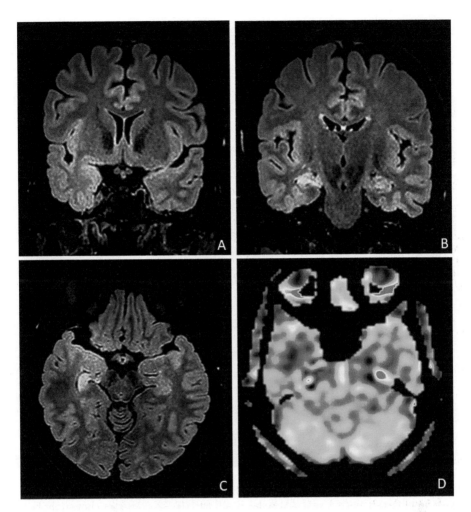

Figure 3.3 Focal cortical dysplasia type 3b: A 26-year-old male presented with seizures since 3 years of age. (**A** and **B**) Coronal FLAIR images show blurring of gray-white matter junction in right anterior temporal lobe, right amygdala with hyperintensity and mild atrophy of right hippocampus. (**C**) Axial FLAIR image shows hyperintensity in right hippocampus and amygdala. (**D**) ASL image shows reduced perfusion in right anterior and medial temporal lobe.

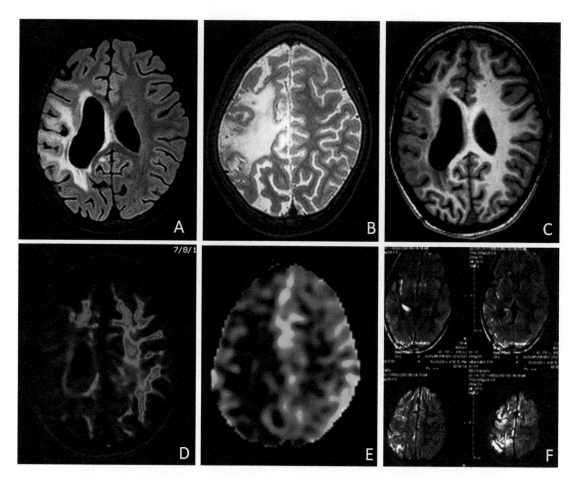

Figure 3.4 Rasmussen encephalitis: A 10-year-old child presented with left focal seizures since 7 years of age and left hemiparesis since 1 year. **(A)** Axial FLAIR and **(B)** T2-w images show right cerebral hemiatrophy with hyperintensities in right fronto-temporo-parieta white matter with dilatation of right lateral ventricle. **(C)** Axial T1-w image shows right hemispheric atrophy with dilatation of right lateral ventricle. **(D)** Axial DTI image shows significant loss of fibers in right cerebral parenchyma. **(E)** ASL shows reduced perfusion in right cerebral parenchyma. **(F)** Old MR performed 2 years back shows FLAIR hyperintensity in right cerebral parenchyma. These lesions have progressed over time resulting in atrophy, with new onset lesions in brain parenchyma which is typical of Rasmussen encephalitis.

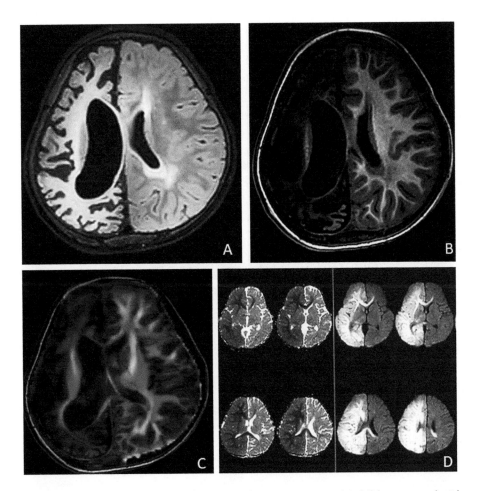

Figure 3.5 Hemiconvulsion hemiplegia epilepsy syndrome: A 3-year-old child presented with progressive left-sided weakness following convulsions 1 month after birth. **(A)** Axial FLAIR and **(B)** T1-w images show right hemispheric atrophy with hyperintensity in subcortical and deep white matter with secondary dilatation of right lateral ventricle. **(C)** Axial DTI shows loss of fibers in right cerebral parenchyma. **(D)** Axial DW MR performed 2 years back had shown uni-hemispheric restricted diffusion following seizures.

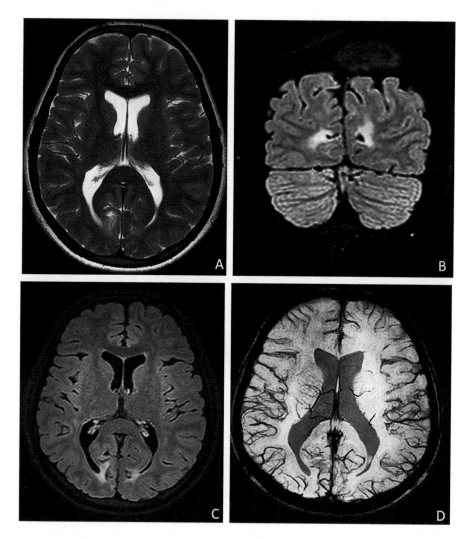

Figure 3.6 Perinatal insult: A 15-year-old boy presented with multiple episodes of seizures since 5 years of age. **(A)** Axial T2, **(B)** FLAIR, and **(C)** coronal FLAIR images show hyperintensity with volume loss involving bilateral occipital lobe subcortical and deep white matter. **(D)** Axial SWI image shows no areas of blooming within the hyperintensity.

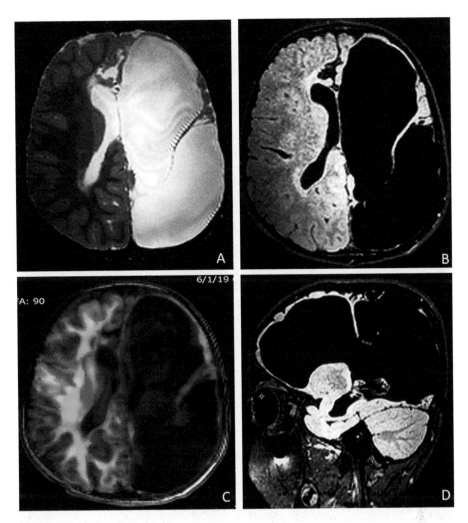

Figure 3.7 Multicystic encephalomalacia: A 7-year-old child presented with seizures since birth and right side weakness. The child also had delayed cry at the time of delivery. **(A)** Axial FLAIR and **(B)** T2-w images show cystic appearing left cerebral parenchyma, showing complete suppression on FLAIR images. **(C)** Axial DTI shows loss of fibers in left cerebral parenchyma. **(D)** Sagittal FLAIR image shows multicystic encephalomalacic changes with preservation of thalamus.

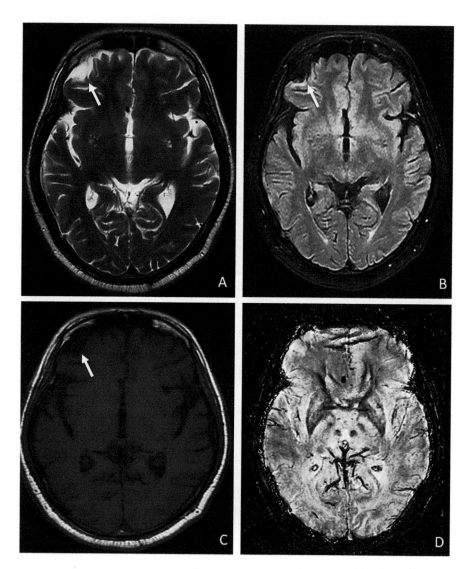

Figure 3.8 Post-traumatic gliosis: A 51-year-old male presented with seizures for the last 1 year. He had severe trauma to the head 2 years back. **(A)** Axial T2 and **(B)** FLAIR images show gliotic changes in right basifrontal lobe (white arrows). **(C)** Axial T-w image shows volume loss in the corresponding region.

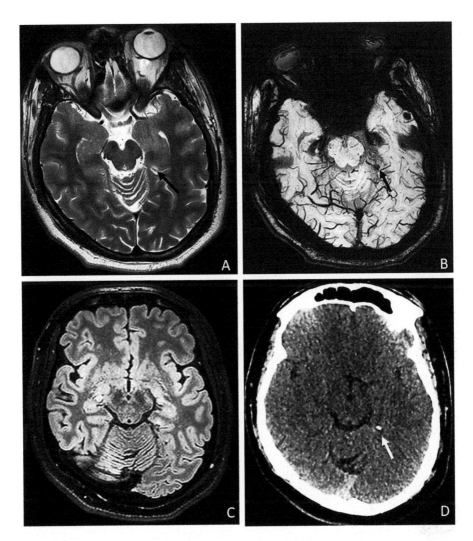

Figure 3.9 Calcified granuloma: A 24-year-old male presented with seizures for the last 2 years. **(A)** Axial T2, **(B)** SWI, and **(C)** FLAIR images show focal hypointensity with blooming in posterior aspect of left parahippocampal gyrus consistent with calcified granuloma (black arrows). **(D)** Axial NCCT confirmed the focal calcification (white arrow).

4

Neurocutaneous syndromes

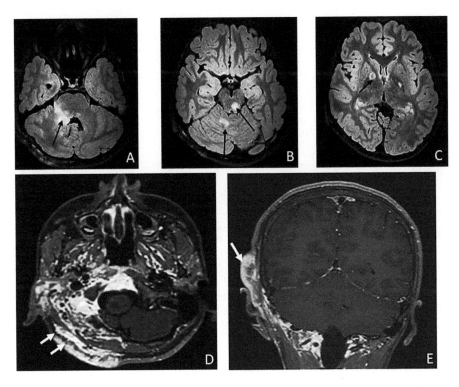

Figure 4.1 Neurofibromatosis (NF) type 1: A 10-year-old child came with multiple swellings on scalp since 8 years. **(A–C)** FLAIR images show multiple hyperintense lesions (arrows) in right middle cerebellar peduncle, dorsal aspect of midbrain and pons, and bilateral globus pallidus likely foci of abnormal signal intensity (FASI). **(D, E)** T1 post gad images show soft tissue thickening and enhancement in right retro-auricular region (thick white arrows) extending into skull base adjacent to jugular foramen indicating plexiform neurofibromas. FASI + plexiform neurofibromas = Neurofibromatosis type 1.

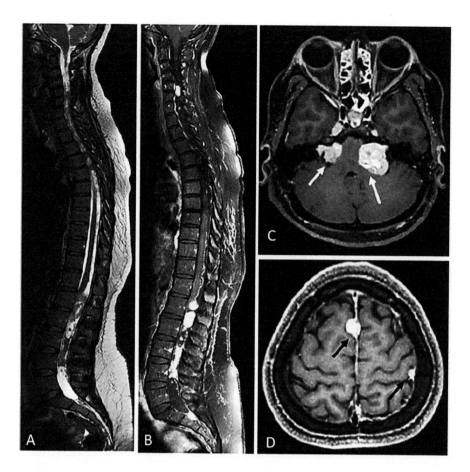

Figure 4.2 Neurofibromatosis (NF) type 2: A 30-year-old female presented with left sided hearing loss and instability of gait since 1 year. **(A)** Sagittal T2 and **(B)** T1-w post-contrast images of spine show multiple enhancing lesions within the spinal canal in cervical, dorsal and lumbar spine suggestive of schwannomas. Axial T1-w post-contrast images **(C, D)** of brain show bilateral acoustic (white arrows) and trigeminal schwannomas with meningiomas (black arrows). Bilateral acoustic schwannomas are diagnostic of NF2.

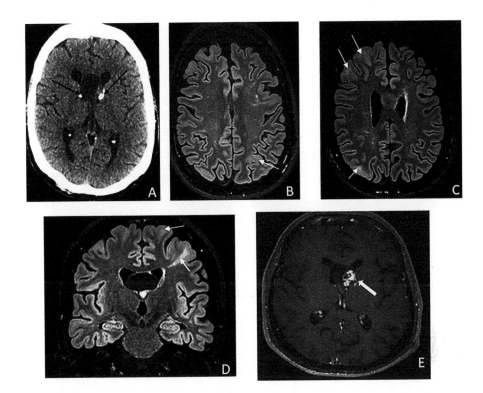

Figure 4.3 Tuberous sclerosis: A 35-year-old patient came with complaints of seizures for past 30 years with headache. **(A)** NCCT shows calcified nodules (arrows) in sub-ependymal region of both lateral ventricles. **(B–D)** MRI FLAIR images show radial bands (thick white arrow in **(D)**) and cortical tubers (arrows) in bilateral fronto-parietal lobes. T1 post gad image **(E)** shows heterogeneously enhancing solid-cystic lesion at foramen of Monro (thick white arrow), suggestive of SEGA (sub-ependymal giant cell astrocytoma). Subependymal nodules + radial bands + cortical tubers + SEGA are consistent with tuberous sclerosis.

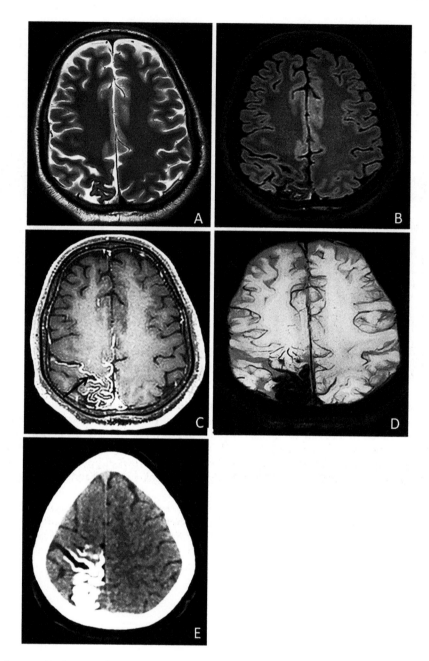

Figure 4.4 Sturge–Weber syndrome: A 30-year-old male presented with left focal seizures and reddish patch in the right side of the forehead. **(A)** Axial T2 and **(B)** FLAIR images show T2 hypo-intensity with gyral atrophy of the cortex in right parietal lobe. **(C)** Axial post contrast image shows leptomeningeal enhancement indicative of multiple pial angiomas in the corresponding region. **(D)** Axial SWI and **(E)** NCCT images show linear gyriform calcification in right parietal lobe with tram track appearance.

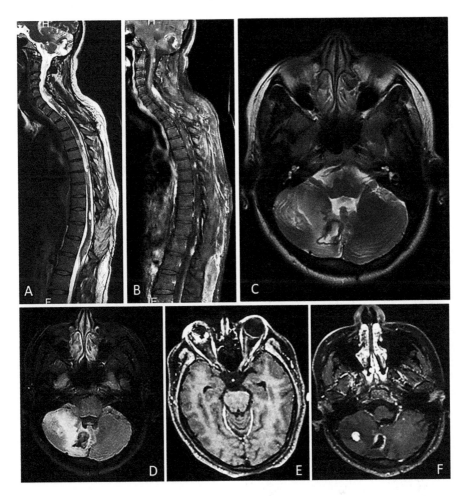

Figure 4.5 Von Hippel–Lindau syndrome: A 30-year-old female presented with left lower limb weakness since 1 year. **(A)** Sagittal T2 and **(B)** T1-w post-contrast images show multiple enhancing lesions in within the cervical and dorsal cord suggestive of hemangioblastomas. **(C)** Axial T2, **(D)** FLAIR, and **(E, F)** T1-w post-contrast images of brain show heterogeneous enhancing lesions in right cerebellar parenchyma suggestive of hemagioblastomas. Note is also made of right orbital hemangioblastoma and secondary pthisis bulbi.

5

Metabolic disorders

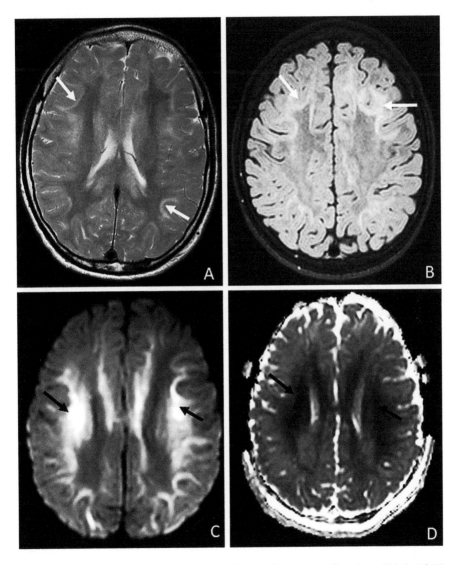

Figure 5.1 Kearns–Sayre syndrome: An 18-year-old boy with status epilepticus. **(A)** Axial T2-w and **(B)** FLAIR images show linear subcortical white matter hyperintensity in supratentorial brain parenchyma (white arrows). **(C)** DWI and **(D)** ADC maps of corresponding areas show hyperintense and hypointense signal respectively, suggestive of diffusion restriction (black arrows).

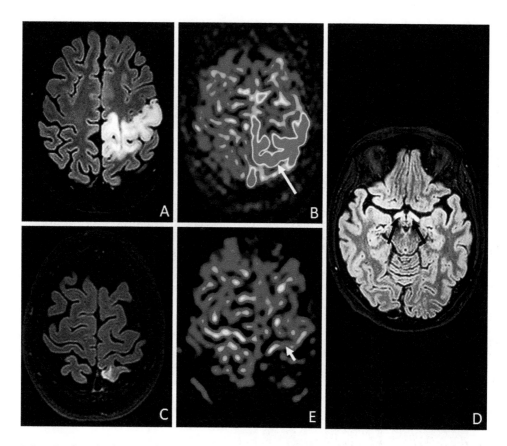

Figure 5.2 Mitochondrial encephalomyopathy, lactic acidosis, and stroke-like episodes (MELAS). A 46-year-old female presented with multiple episodes of relapsing and remitting focal neurological deficits since 6 years. **(A)** Axial FLAIR image taken at the time of an event shows focal hyperintense signal involving both grey and white matter of left precentral gyrus. **(B)** Corresponding areas in perfusion-weighted images show increased perfusion (white long arrow). **(D)** Axial FLAIR image at the level of midbrain shows hyperintense signal involving both proximal optic tracts (black arrows). **(C)** Axial FLAIR and **(E)** perfusion-weighted image performed 6 months later show near complete resolution of changes seen previously (white short arrow).

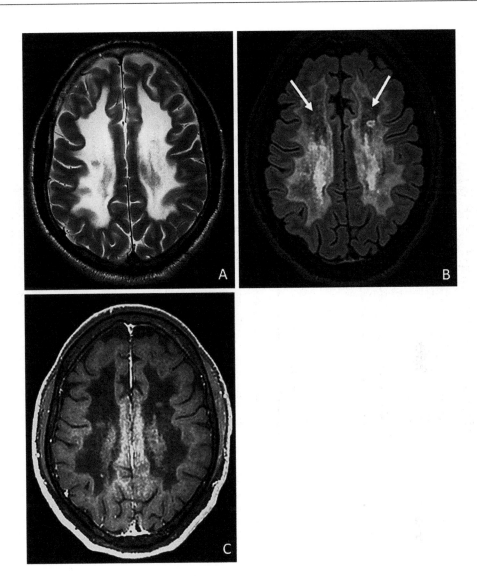

Figure 5.3 Vanishing white matter disease: **(A)** Axial T2-w image shows confluent hyperintense signal involving supratentorial deep and periventricular white matter. **(B)** Axial FLAIR image shows predominantly hyperintense signal with few areas of fluid suppression appearing as dark areas, suggestive of cystic changes (white arrows). **(C)** Axial T1-w post-gadolinium image shows no enhancement.

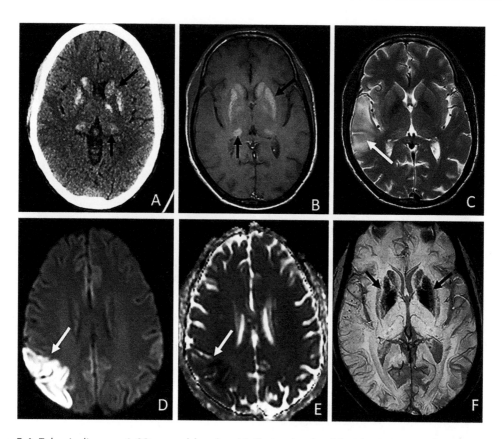

Figure 5.4 Fabry's disease: A 29-year-old male with first episode of focal seizures 15 days back.
(A) Axial NCCT image of the brain shows calcifications involving bilateral basal ganglia and thalami.
(B) Axial T1 and (C) T2-w images show hyperintense basal ganglia and thalami, with corresponding areas showing blooming in (D) axial SWI, consistent with calcifications (black arrows). Right parietal lobe shows a focal area of hyperintense signal involving both grey and white matter in Axial T2-w image, which shows hyperintense and hypointense signals in (E) DWI and (F) ADC map respectively, suggestive of diffusion restriction and consistent with acute infarct (white arrows).

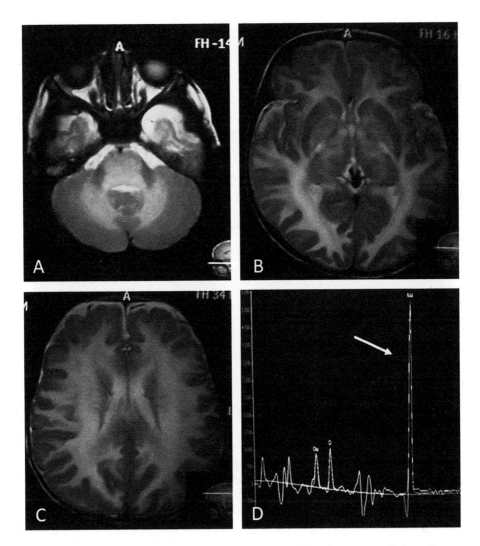

Figure 5.5 Canavan's Disease: MR imaging in a 2-year-old child with macrocephaly and developmental delay. (A–C) MR images show diffuse white matter hyperintensities involving cerebral and cerebellar white matter, and descending tracts. (D) MRS shows a large N-acetyl aspartate peak (arrow). These image findings are characteristic of Canavan's disease.

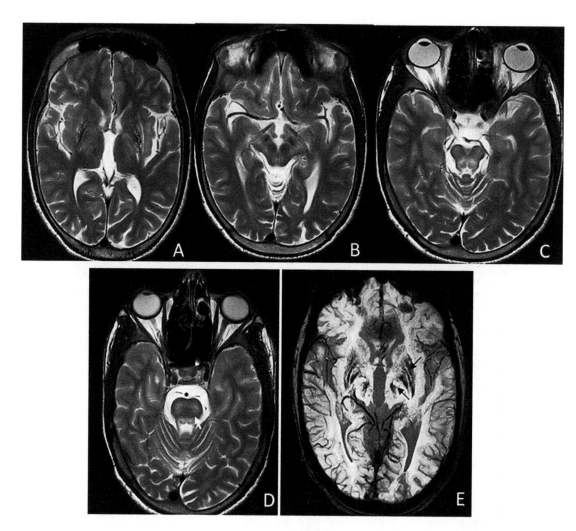

Figure 5.6 Wilson's disease: A 20-year-old patient presented with dystonia and parkinsonian features. Examination revealed KF ring in his both eyes. **(A)** MRI reveals abnormal T2 hyperintensity in bilateral lentiform nucleus, **(B–D)** midbrain, peri-aqueductal white matter and pons with relative sparing of red nucleus (giant panda sign). **(E)** Abnormal blooming is seen in bilateral lentiform nucleus and substantia nigra. Image findings are consistent with Wilson's disease, which is a disorder of copper metabolism.

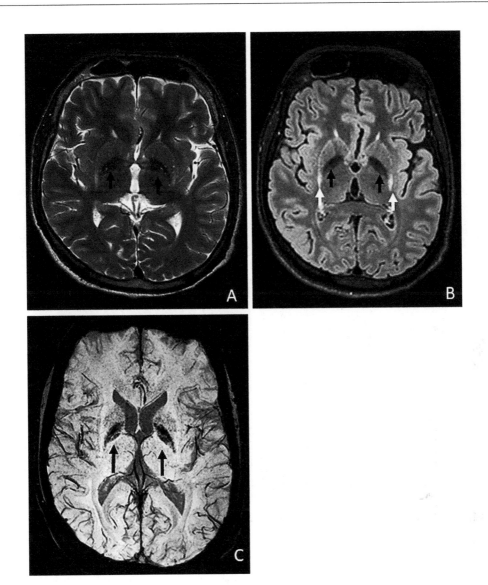

Figure 5.7 Neurodegeneration with brain iron accumulation: A 19-year-old boy presented with dystonia of upper limbs for last 6 years. **(A)** Axial T2-w and **(B)** FLAIR image shows hypointense signal in the globus pallidus, consistent with heavy metal deposition (black short arrows). Hyperintense signal is seen in the lateral and posterior margin of putamen (white arrows). **(C)** Axial SWI image shows hypointense signal (blooming) in the region corresponding to the globus pallidus, consistent with metal deposition disease (black long arrows).

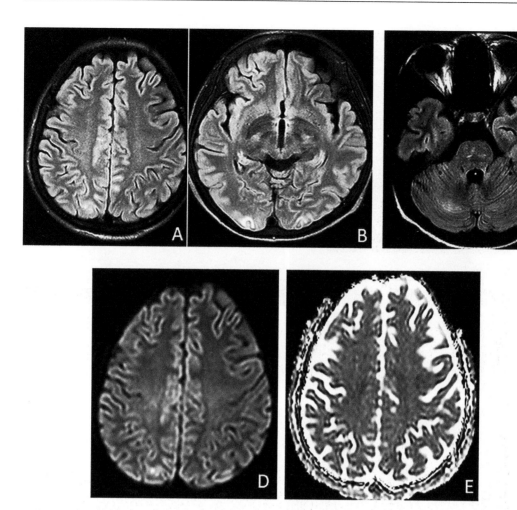

Figure 5.8 Posterior reversible encephalopathy syndrome (PRES): A 21-year-old known sickle cell patient came with complains of multiple episodes of seizures in post-partum period. **(A–E)** MRI shows abnormal symmetrical FLAIR hyperintensity in bilateral pareito-occiptial lobes subcortical white matter, right cerebellar white matter with focal area of diffusion restriction in right parietal lobe. Note is made of white matter changes in central aspect of the pons. PRES predominantly involves subcortical white matter of both parietooccipital lobe without showing restricted diffusion.

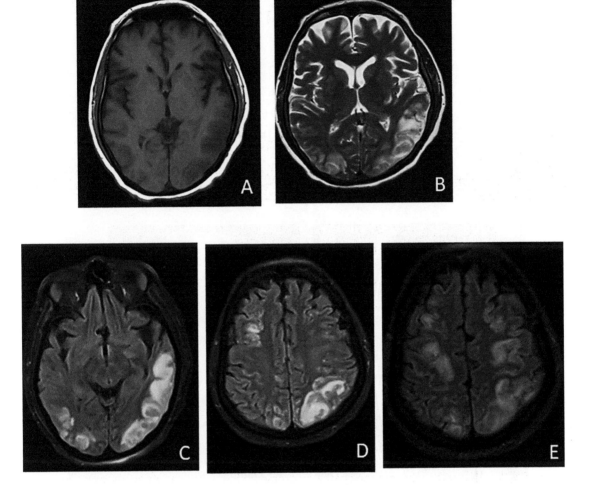

Figure 5.9 Another typical case of PRES. This patient was a 62-year-old man with chronic kidney disease who presented with accelerated hypertension and altered sensorium.

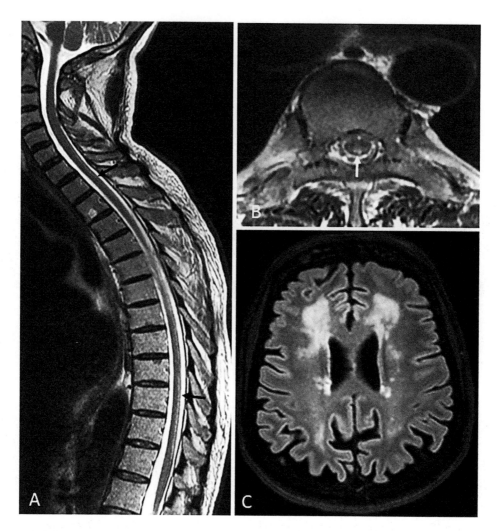

Figure 5.10 Subacute combined degeneration of the cord (SACD): A 51-year-old male presented with rapidly progressive dementia. **(A)** Sagittal T2-w image of cervico-dorsal spine shows long segment intramedullary, hyperintensity is seen in posterior column of the cord in cervical and dorsal region (black arows). **(B)** Axial T2-w image at the level of dorsal spine shows hyperintensity in both posterior columns with inverted rabbit ear sign (white arrows). **(C)** Axial FLAIR image shows confluent and few discrete hyperintensities in both frontal and parietal lobe white matter. This is one of the treatable cause of dementia with good outcome.

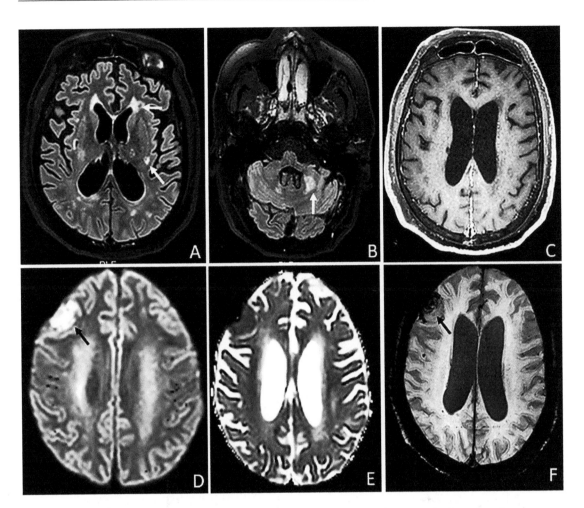

Figure 5.11 Cocaine leukoencephalopathy: A 46-year-old male with history of substance abuse (cocaine) since 15 year of age, presented with difficulty in walking. **(A)** Axial FLAIR images show multiple discrete hyperintensities in both frontal and parietal lobe white matter, posterior aspect of both putamen and deep cerebellar white matter (white arrows). **(B)** Axial T1-w image after contrast administration shows no enhancement. **(C)** Axial DWI and **(D)** ADC images show no restricted diffusion in the white matter lesions. **(E)** Axial SWI image shows punctate blooming in right frontal subcortical white matter. **(F)** Note is made of an incidental meningioma in right frontal lobe convexity (black arrow).

6

Demyelination and inflammatory disorders

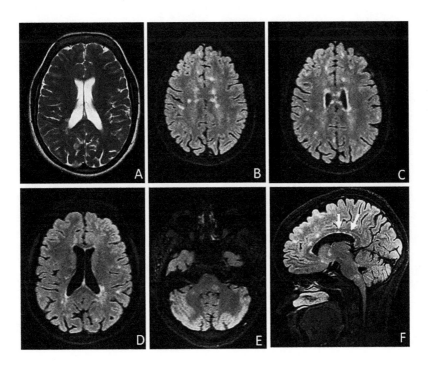

Figure 6.1 Multiple sclerosis (MS): A 23-year-old lady presented with multiple neurological deficits over the past 3 years. **(A–E)** Axial T2 and FLAIR images show multiple small white matter lesions distributed in juxtacortical, periventricular and infratentorial brain parenchyma. **(F)** Sag FLAIR image shows multiple white matter lesions in the callososeptal interface (white arrow).

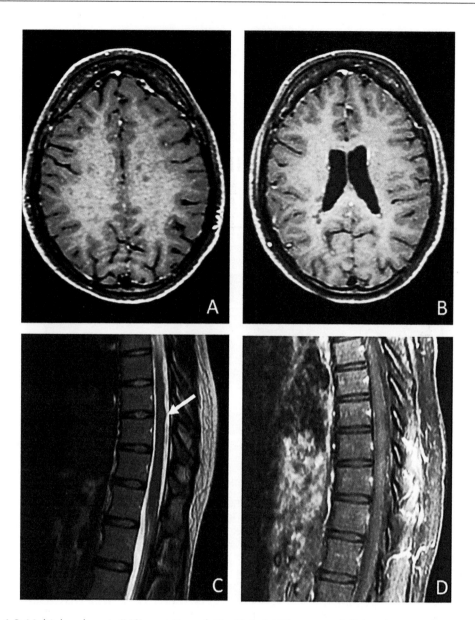

Figure 6.2 Multiple sclerosis (MS) – continued: **(A, B)** Axial T1 post-gadolinium images show no enhancement. **(C)** Saggital T2-w image of the dorsal cord shows a single short segment cord hyperintensity (white arrow), which is not showing any enhancement in the **(D)** sagittal T1 post-gadolinium image. MS is the commonest primary demyelinating disorder in adults.

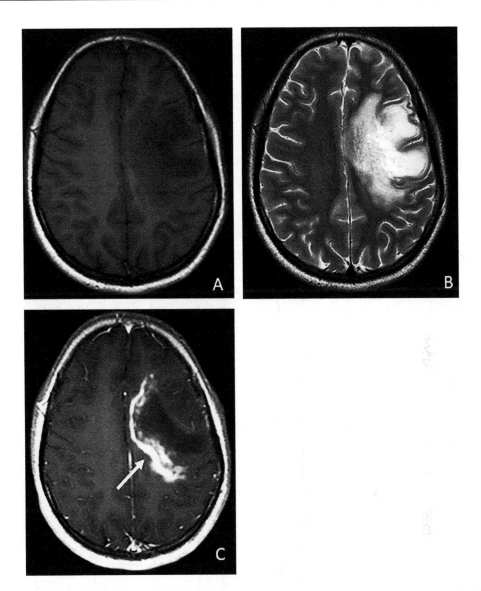

Figure 6.3 Tumefactive demyelination: A 16-year-old girl presented with acute onset speech difficulty and right-sided weakness. **(A)** Axial T1-w image shows confluent hypointense lesion involving white matter of left frontal lobe. **(B)** It appears hyperintense in axial T2-w image. **(C)** Axial T1 post-gadolinium images show thick linear enhancement along the medial margin of the lesion (white arrow). No mass effect is evident.

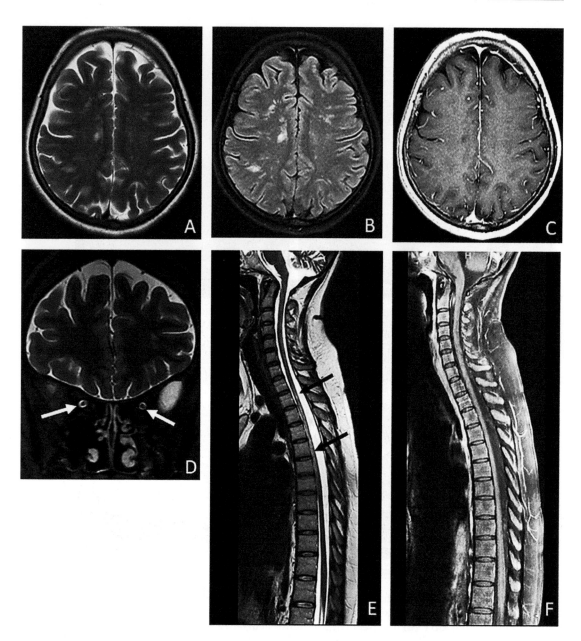

Figure 6.4 Neuromyelitis optica: A 22-year-old female presented with acute onset paraparesis with an old history of visual loss that has recovered partially. **(A)** Axial T2-w and **(B)** FLAIR images show multiple small hyperintense lesions involving subcortical and deep-white matter of centrum semiovale on both sides. **(C)** Axial T1 post-gadolinium image shows no enhancement. **(D)** Coronal T2 images show optic nerve atrophy on both sides with prominent CSF spaces (white arrows). Left optic nerve also shows hyperintense signal, suggestive of optic neuritis. **(E)** Sagittal T2-w image of the spine shows long segment hyperintensity of the upper dorsal cord (black arrows). **(F)** Sagittal T1-w post-gadolinium image shows no enhancement.

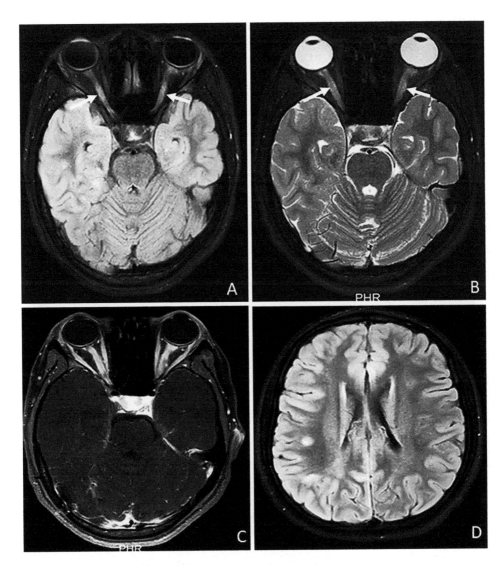

Figure 6.5 Anti-myelin oligodendrocyte glycoprotein (MOG) associated demyelination: A 14-year-old female presented with sequential loss of vision in both eyes. **(A)** Axial T2 and **(B)** FLAIR images show long segment hyperintensity with thickening of intraorbital segment of both optic nerves. **(C)** Axial post-contrast images showed enhancement of both optic nerves and perioptic sheaths. **(D)** Axial FLAIR image also shows few discrete hyperintensities in right frontal and parietal lobe white matter.

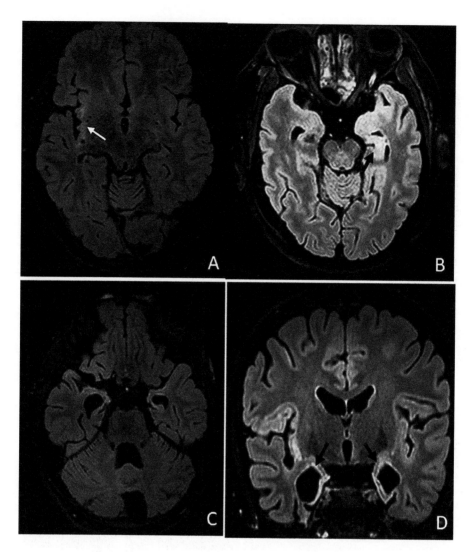

Figure 6.6 Autoimmune encephalitis: A 45-year-old lady presented with dysarthria and gait ataxia with behavioral change for past 9 months. **(A–C)** Axial and **(D)** coronal FLAIR images shows hyperintensity in bilateral hippocampus (black arrows), both medial temporal lobes and insular cortex (white arrow) along with atrophy of hippocampus and anteromedial temporal lobes. Autoimmune encephalitis characteristically involves both temporal lobes and insular cortex.

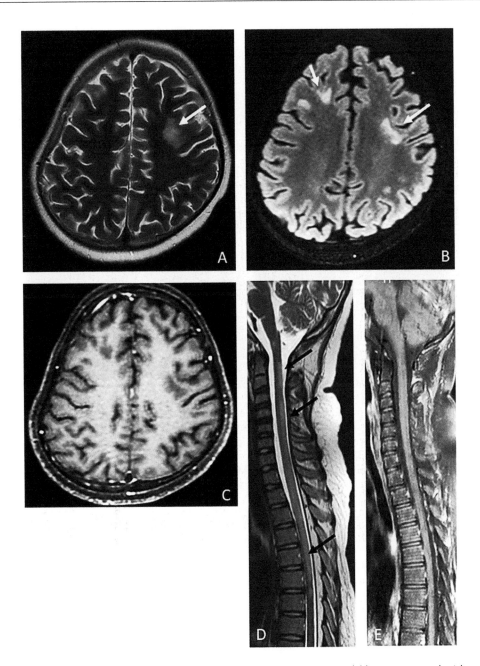

Figure 6.7 Acute demyelinating encephalomyelitis (ADEM): A 13-year-old boy presented with acute onset quadriparesis with bladder and bowel involvement. (A) Axial T2-w and (B) FLAIR images show multiple flame-shaped hyperintensities (white arrows), involving the subcortical white matter. (C) Axial T1 post-gadolinium image shows no enhancement. (D) Saggital T2-w image of spine shows multiple long and short segment cord hyperintensities (black arrows), not showing any enhancement in (E) saggital T1 post-gadolinium image. The clinical setting and imaging findings are consistent with ADEM.

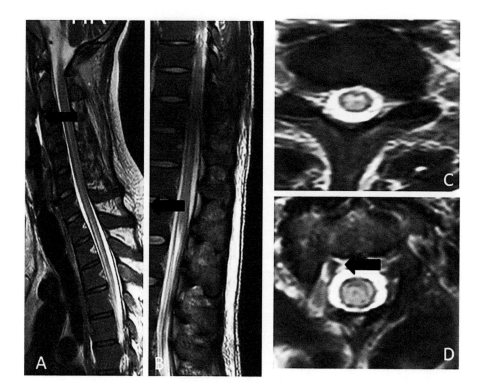

Figure 6.8 Acute transverse myelitis (ATM): A 30-year-old male patient presented with complaints of bilateral lower limb weakness and urinary retention for past 2 weeks. **(A, B)** MRI sagittal T2-w image of cervical and lumbar spine reveals long segment intramedullary hyperintensity within the spinal cord involving the conus. **(C, D)** Axial T2-w image of cervical spine shows central intramedullary hyperintensity with mild expansion of the cord. ATM usually involves long segment of the cord (> 2-vertebral body segments) with involvement of the central aspect of the cord.

Neurovascular diseases

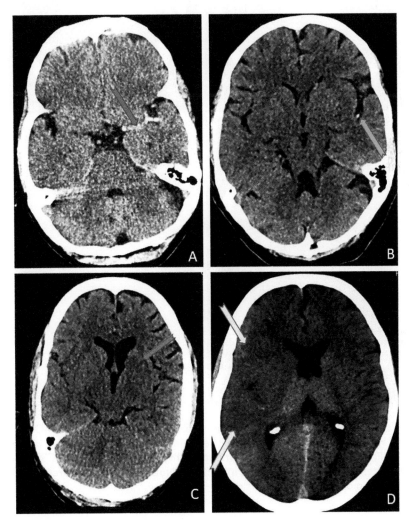

Figure 7.1 Hyperacute infarct: In a patient with suspected acute stroke undergoing non-contrast CT, it is very crucial to recognise some subtle signs which are highly specific for ischemic stroke and can manifest within a few hours. **(A)** NCCT brain shows (arrow) a linear hyperdense structure in left Sylvian fissure which represents M1 segment of left middle cerebral artery (Hyperdense MCA sign) indicating acute thrombus within the artery. **(B)** Similarly the arrow represents clot within one of the divisions of MCA and is called MCA dot sign. **(C)** Arrow shows margins of left lentiform nucleus being indistinct with blurring of left basal ganglia (blue arrow). **(D)** Loss of grey and white matter differentiation in right MCA territory in a different patient (yellow arrow).

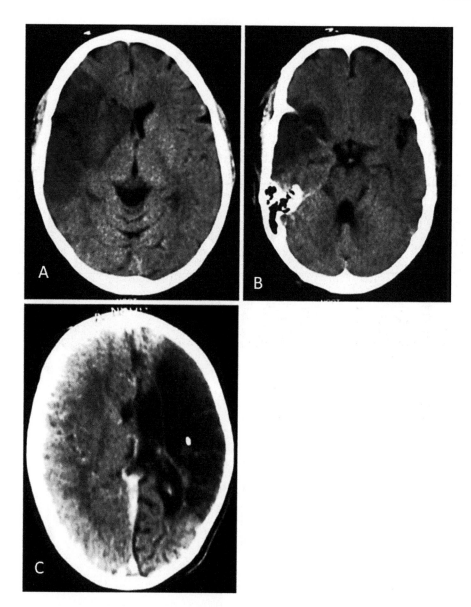

Figure 7.2 Stroke: **(A, B)** NCCT scan shows wedge-shaped hypodensity in right MCA territory s/o acute infarct. Hypodensity is a sign of established infarct. With time, infarcted tissue undergo volume loss and gliotic change, resulting in pronounced hypodensity (similar to CSF) and dilatation of adjacent sulcal spaces and ventricles (chronic infarct). **(C)** Note the chronic infarct involving left MCA territory with dilatation of left lateral ventricle.

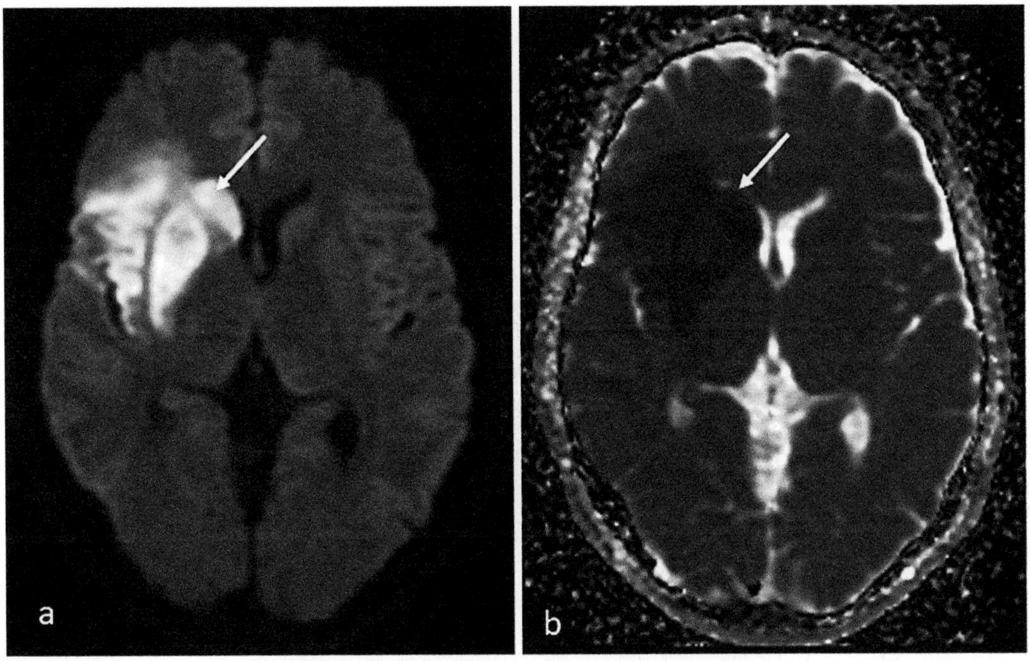

Figure 7.3 Stroke: Axial DWI **(A)** and ADC **(B)** images show restricted diffusion in the right lentiform nucleus, insular cortex and right frontal operculum, corresponding to low ADC value in ADC (white arrow in **(A** and **B)**) s/o acute infarct. Restricted diffusion can be seen within 30 minutes after stroke and found positive in approximately 95% of cases.

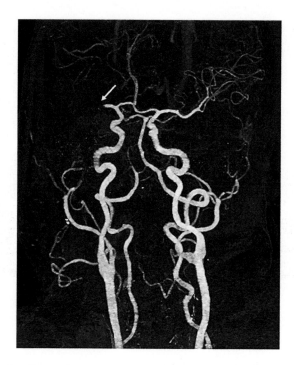

Figure 7.4 CT angiography: Coronal maximum intensity projection (MIP) image shows abrupt cutoff in right M1 MCA (white arrow) s/o thrombosis. It is important to detect this as it implies that the patient is a potential candidate for mechanical thrombectomy.

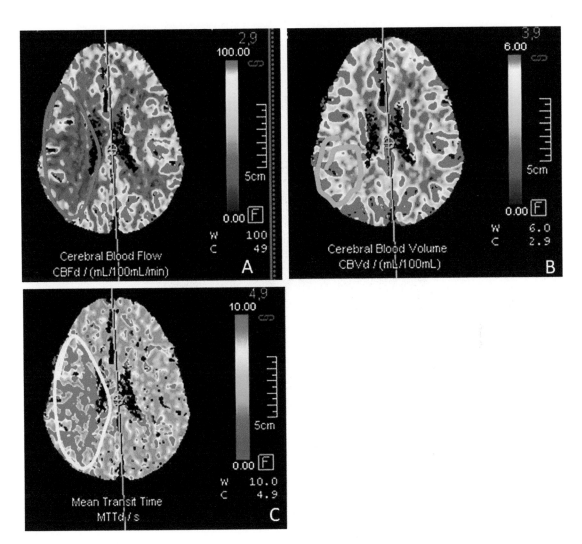

Figure 7.5 CT Perfusion: CT perfusion is performed in acute ischemic stroke to identify infarct core and salvageable tissue, hence play an important role in deciding whether a patient would benefit from mechanical thrombectomy in a case of large vessel occlusion. (A–C) Cerebral blood volume map shows regions with low blood volume, which indicate infarct core (marked as green region in CBV map). Cerebral blood flow is reduced in both infarct core and salvageable tissue (marked as red in CBF map). Similarly, mean transit time is also increased in both infarct core and salvageable tissue (marked as yellow in MTT map). A mismatch of CBF & CBV map or MTT & CBV map indicates the presence of salvageable tissue, otherwise called as 'penumbra' that can be saved by reperfusion.

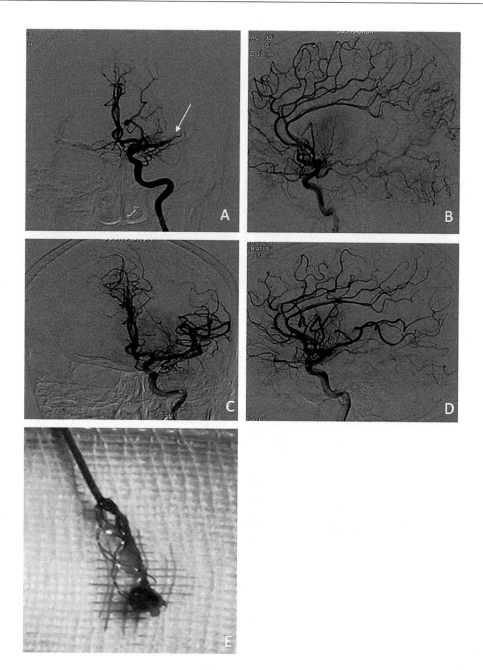

Figure 7.6 Mechanical thrombectomy: A 56-year-old male presented with sudden onset weakness in left side with aphasia for 4 hours. **(A, B)** DSA AP and lateral view show non visualization of left MCA M2 segments with cutoff at mid M1 (white arrow). **(C, D)** Post procedure control angiogram showed complete recanalization of MCA and its branches. **(E)** Clot within the stent after post procedure.

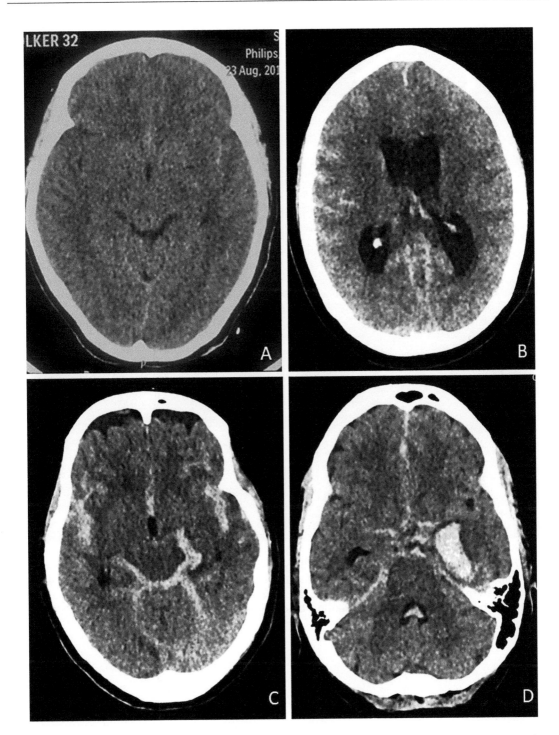

Figure 7.7 Subarachnoid hemorrhage (SAH) – Fisher grading: Axial NCCT images show various Fisher grades of SAH. **(A)** Thin SAH in the anterior interhemispheric fissure and left Sylvian fissure (Fisher 1), **(B)** diffuse thin SAH with hydrocephlaus (Fisher 2), **(C)** diffuse thick SAH (Fisher 3) and **(D)** SAH with intraparenchymal hemorrhage (Fisher 4).

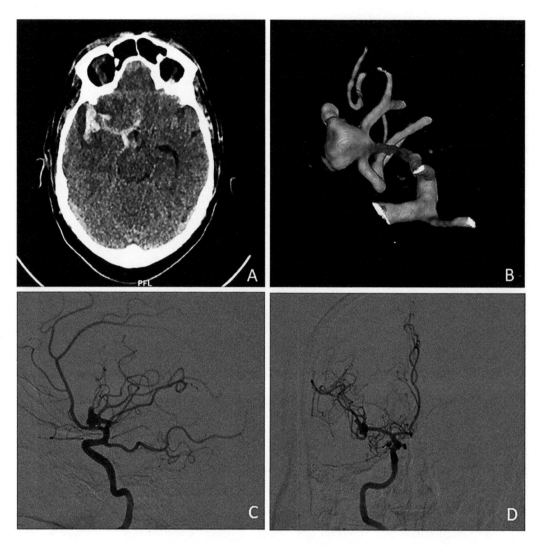

Figure 7.8 Middle cerebral artery aneurysm: A 54-year-old man presented with severe headache and loss of consciousness 2 days back. **(A, B)** NCCT scan shows acute bleed in right temporal lobe with SAH basal cistern and right ambient cistern. **(C, D)** 3D image and right ICA DSA run shows aneurysm in right MCA bifurcation (white arrow). Sentinel bleed identifies possible site of aneurysm.

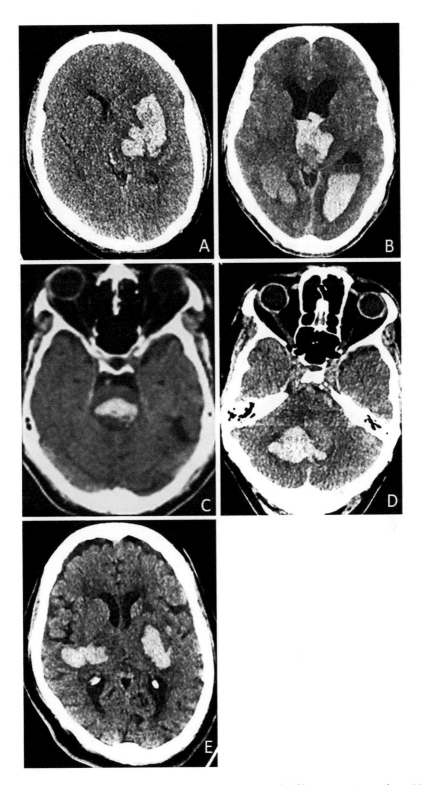

Figure 7.9 Intracerebral hemorrhage (ICH): Axial NCCT scans of different patients show **(A)** acute bleed in left external capsule, **(B)** left thalamus with intraventricular extension, **(C)** central aspect of pons, **(D)** right cerebellar parenchyma, **(E)** posterior aspect of both putamen. These are the typical sites of hypertensive bleed in the brain.

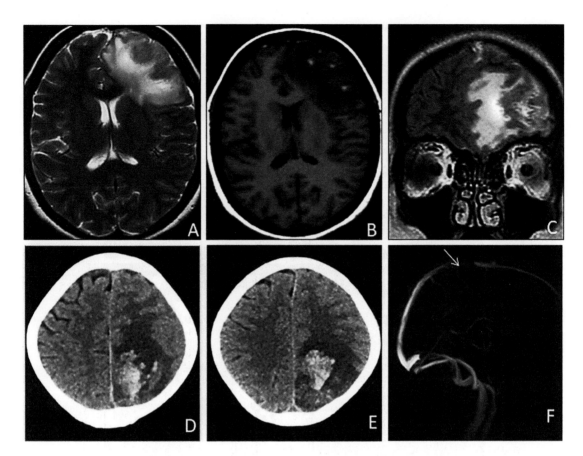

Figure 7.10 Central vein thrombosis (CVT): A 24-year-old female presented with headache with blurring of vision for 3 days. (A, B) Axial T2 and T1 images show bleed with adjacent perilesional edema in left anterior and superior frontal lobe. (C) Coronal T2 image showing bleed in left anterior and superior frontal lobe. (D–E) NCCT scan shows bleed in left parietal lobe with hyperdense superior sagittal sinus. (F) MRV MIP image shows filling defect in middle part of superior sagittal sinus s/o thrombosis. Infarct with hemorrhage not corresponding to any arterial territory is a clue for the diagnosis of CVT.

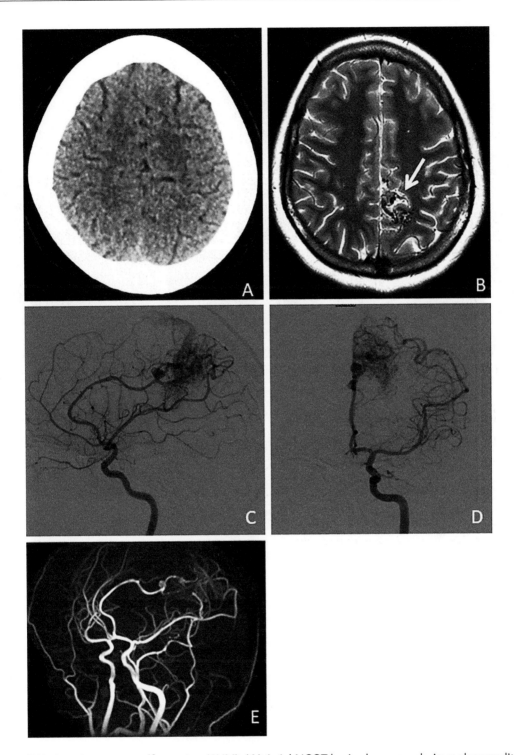

Figure 7.11 Arteriovenous malformation (AVM): **(A)** Axial NCCT brain shows no obvious abnormality. **(B)** Multiple serpiginious vessels are seen in precuneus region of left parietal lobe, suggestive of nidus (white arrow). **(C, D)** PA and lateral projection of left ICA angiogram show nidus in the left posteiror pericallosal region, supplied by left pericallosal artery and a branch of left MCA, drained by a large vein into superior sagittal sinus. **(E)** TOF MRA shows identical findings.

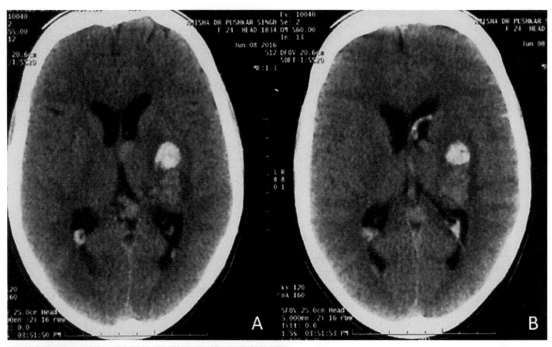

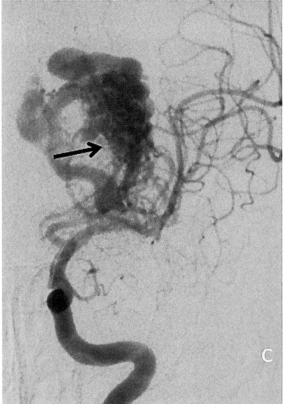

Figure 7.12 Ruptured arteriovenous malformation (AVM): **(A, B)** Acute intraparenchymal hemorrhage is seen in the left lentiform nucleus, which is otherwise a typical site for hypertensive hemorrhage. **(C)** PA projection of left internal carotid angiogram shows parenchymal AVM (black arrow) with feeders from lenticulostriate branches of left MCA.

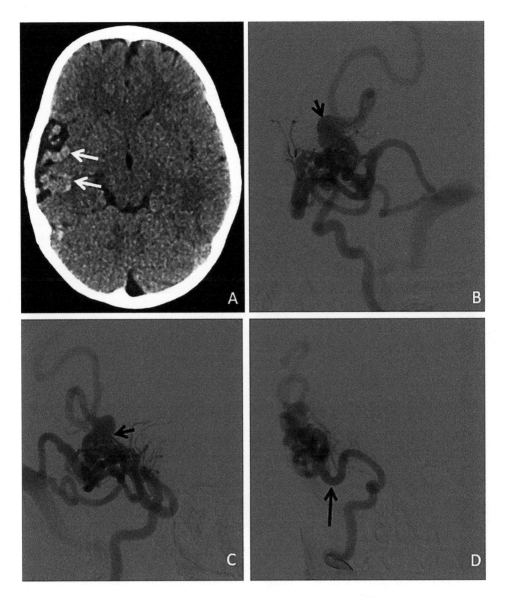

Figure 7.13 Pial arteriovenous fistula (AVF): **(A)** Axial NCCT image shows focal area of volume loss in the right temporal region, with multiple serpiginious vessels (white arrows). **(B–D)** PA and oblique projections of right ICA angiogram show hypertrophied right MCA (long black arrow) directly opening into dilated venous sac (short black arrow), which eventually drains into right transverse sinus and superior sagittal sinus.

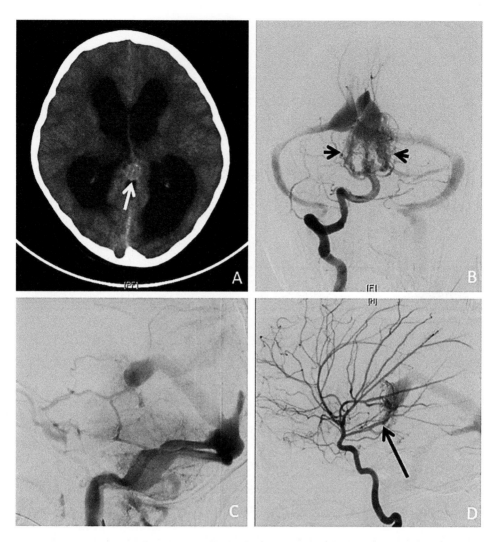

Figure 7.14 Vein of Galen malformation: **(A)** Axial NCCT image shows hydrocephalus. Note the rounded hyperdense structure which represents venous sac (white arrow). **(B, C)** AP and lateral projections of vertebral angiogram show multiple hypertrophied posterior choroidal feeders (black short arrows) draining into a dilated sac which in turn drains into straight sinus. **(D)** ICA angiogram shows hypertrophied anterior choroidal feeders (black long arrows) opening directly into the sac.

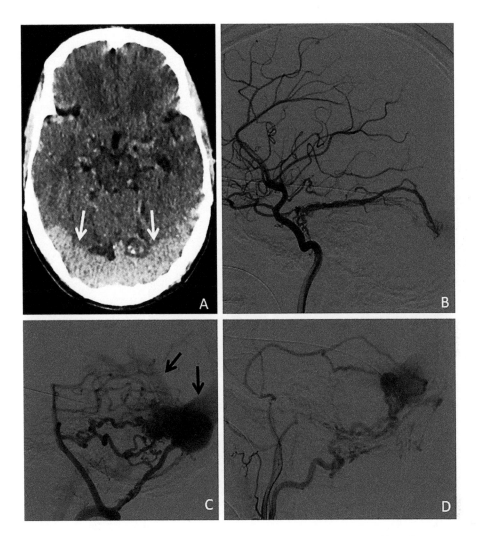

Figure 7.15 Dural arteriovenous fistula (DAVF): **(A)** Axial NCCT image shows dilated transverse sinuses (white arrows) and multiple prominent vessels in the basal cisterns. **(B–D)** Lateral projections of internal carotid artery, vertebral artery, and external carotid artery angiograms show multiple arterial feeders from meningeal branches of internal carotid artery, posterior meningeal artery, anterior inferior cerebellar artery, middle meningeal, occipital and ascending pharyngeal artery, draining directly into dilated transverse sinuses with reflux (black arrow).

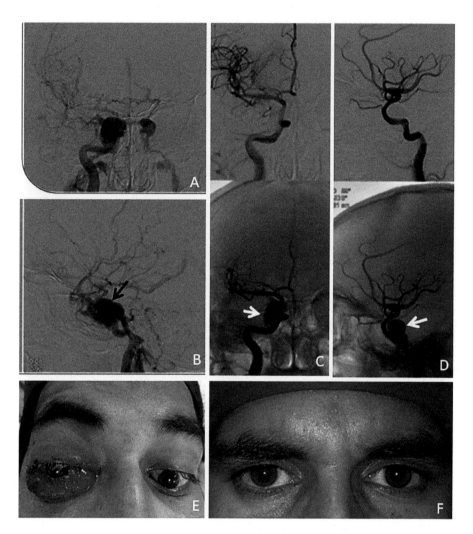

Figure 7.16 Carotid-cavernous fistula (CCF): **(A–D)** PA and lateral projection of right CCA angiograms show caroticocavernous fistula, evidenced by direct opening of cavernous carotid artery into dilated cavernous sinus (black arrow) with cortical venous reflux. Post-embolization with detachable balloon (white arrows) shows complete obliteration of fistula. **(E–F)** Clinical photograph shows proptosis and redness in the right eye, which resolved completely post-procedure.

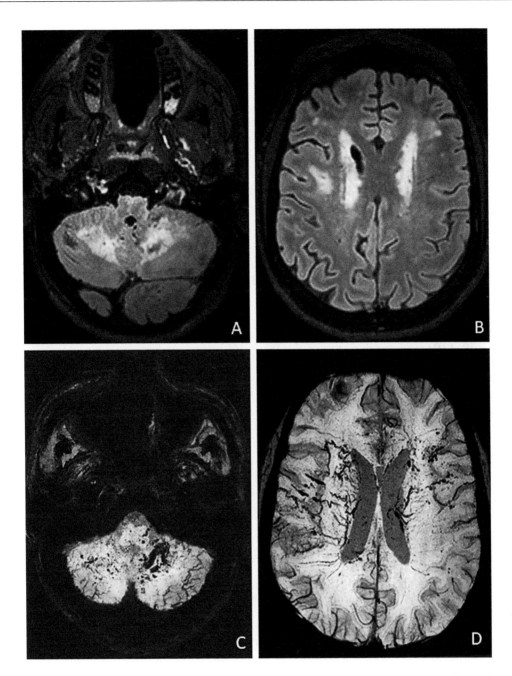

Figure 7.17 Vasculitis: A 25-year-old male presented with headache and recurrent neurological deficits for last 6 months. **(A)** Axial FLAIR shows multiple confluent and discrete hyperintensities in both cerebellar parenchyma and **(B)** frontoparietal lobe white matter. **(C)** SWI images show multiple foci of blooming in both cerebellar and **(D)** cerebral parenchyma with corkscrewing of vessels. SWI blooming in both MCA territories and both cerebellar parenchyma are imaging features classical of vasculitis.

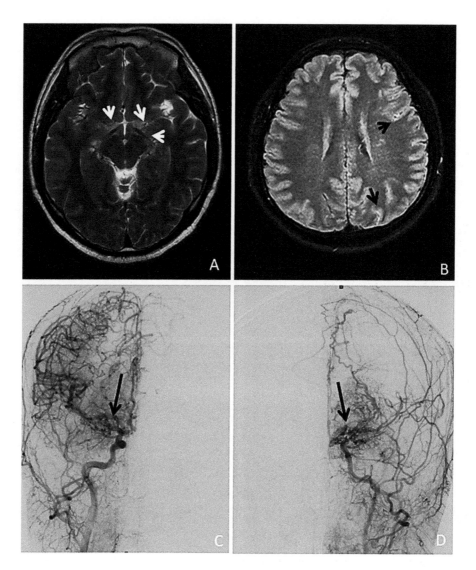

Figure 7.18 Moyamoya disease: **(A)** Axial T2-w image shows multiple small flow voids in the CSF spaces of basal cisterns (white short arrows). **(B)** Multiple linear hyperintense signals are seen in the frontoparietal sulci in FLAIR images, that correspond the slow collateral flow, termed as 'ivy' sign (black short arrows). **(C, D)** PA projections of right and left common carotid artery angiograms show severe narrowing of both terminal internal carotid arteries with 'puff of smoke' like basal collaterals (long black arrows) reforming distal vessels.

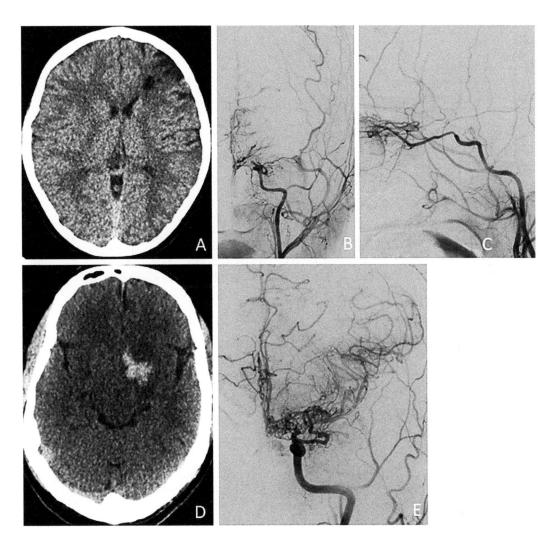

Figure 7.19 Moyamoya disease – continued: Moyamoya disease can present with seizures, infarcts or hemorrhages. Upper panel shows a patient who presented with infarct. **(A)** Axial NCCT image shows chronic infarct in left frontal external watershed zone. **(B)** PA and **(C)** lateral projections left CCA angiograms show near complete narrowing of left terminal internal carotid artery beyond the origin of ophthalmic artery. **(D)** (another patient) Intraparenchymal hemorrhage due to rupture of one of the dysplastic basal collaterals. **(E)** PA projection of left CCA angiogram shows severe narrowing of left terminal ICA with hypertrophied basal collaterals.

8

Central nervous system tumors

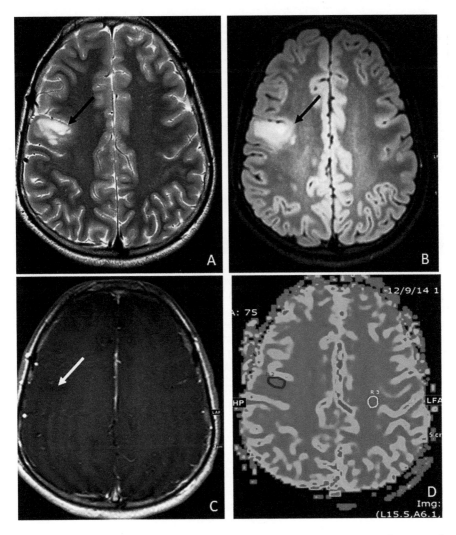

Figure 8.1 Low-grade glioma: A 34-year-old male presented with complex partial seizures for the last 1 year. **(A)** Axial T2 and **(B)** FLAIR images show a well-defined, bright, subcortical lesion (black arrows) in the right posterior frontal region without perilesional edema. **(C)** No enhancement (white arrow), or **(D)** increase in perfusion is noted. Common low-grade gliomas causing epilepsy are ganglioglioma and DNET, followed by oligodendroglioma and diffuse astrocytoma. Here the likely diagnosis is astrocytoma by virtue of subcortical location, for the others mentioned above are cortical tumors.

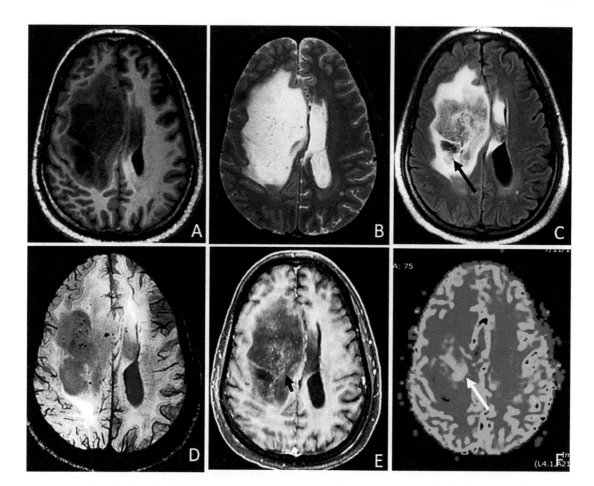

Figure 8.2 Anaplastic astrocytoma: A 45-year-old woman presented with seizures for the past 3 years and recent left sided weakness. **(A)** Axial T1 and **(B)** T2-w images show a large, diffuse, white matter centered mass lesion, which is bright in T2 and dark in T1. **(C)** Axial FLAIR images show suppression at few areas (long black arrow), suggesting cystic nature. **(D)** Axial SWI show few punctate black dots, representing areas of hemorrhages. **(E)** Axial T1 post-contrast image shows subtle enhancement in the lesion (black short arrow), with corresponding areas showing **(F)**, increased perfusion (white arrow). Hemorrhage, enhancement, and increased perfusion are signs of higher grade in a glioma.

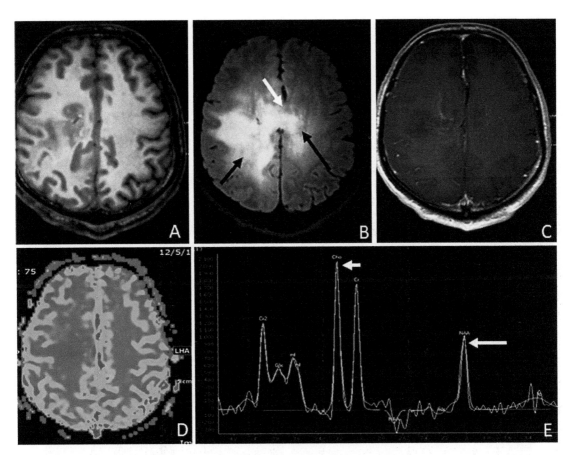

Figure 8.3 Gliomatosis: A 34-year-old female presented with altered behavior for the past 3 months
(A) Axial T1 and **(B)** FLAIR image shows diffuse and confluent white matter lesion which is bright
in FLAIR (black arrows). **(C)** Note that the lesion is spreading to the other hemisphere through the
corpus callosum (white arrow). Post contrast, most of the lesion shows no enhancement. **(D)** Perfusion
image shows no increased perfusion. Absence of any significant enhancement and reduced perfusion
indicate low grade of the tumor. **(E)** MR spectroscopy shows elevated choline peak (short white arrow)
and a fall in NAA peak (long white arrow) which is commonly seen in glioma. The term gliomatosis
is done away with in the recent WHO-2016 classification and the entity is called simply as diffuse
astrocytoma.

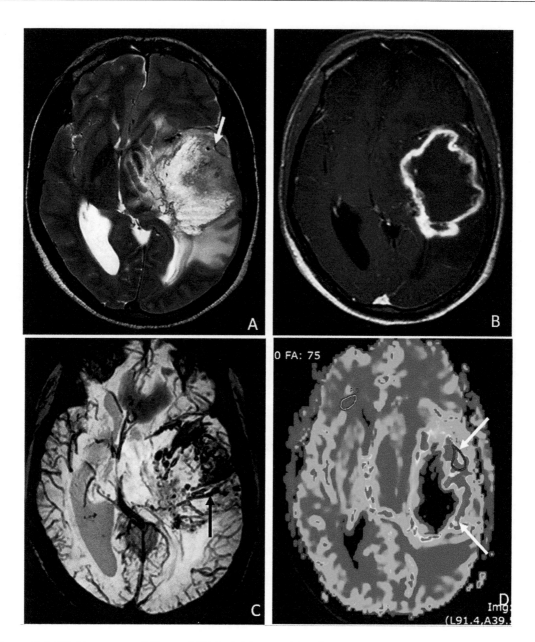

Figure 8.4 Glioblastoma multiforme (GBM): A 52-year-old male presented with 2 months of headache. **(A)** A large heterogeneous mass lesion is seen in the left temporal and insular region with mass effect and perilesional edema in T2-w image. Note neovascularization, seen as dark flow voids (short white arrows). **(B)** Axial T1 post-contrast image shows thick rim enhancement, with central non-enhancing necrotic areas. **(C)** Axial SWI shows extensive dark areas suggestive of hemorrhages (black arrow). **(D)** Perfusion image shows increased perfusion in the rim (long white arrows). Neovascularity, hemorrhage, and necrosis are hallmarks of GBM.

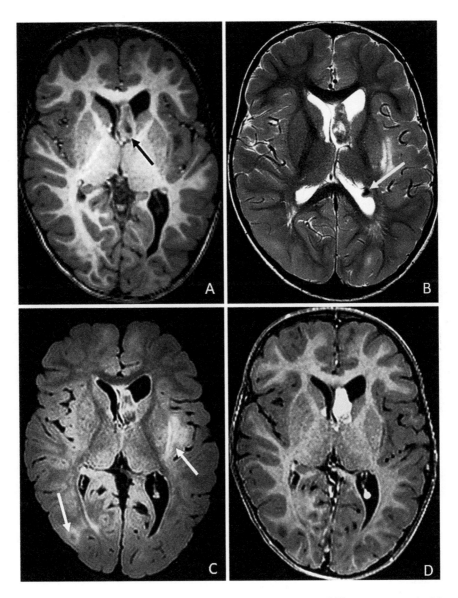

Figure 8.5 Subependymal giant cell astrocytoma (SEGA): A 12-year-old boy presented with seizures since 2 years of age. **(A)** Axial T1, **(B)** T2, and **(C, D)** FLAIR images show an ovoid heterogeneous lesion in the left foramen of Monro, projecting into the frontal horn of left lateral ventricle (black arrow). It shows homogeneous and intense enhancement, after contrast administration. Note the multiple tubers in left insula and right occipital lobe (white arrows) and a calcified subependymal nodule in left atrium (yellow arrow). SEGA, subependymal nodules, radial lines, and cortical tubers are characteristic findings of tuberous sclerosis.

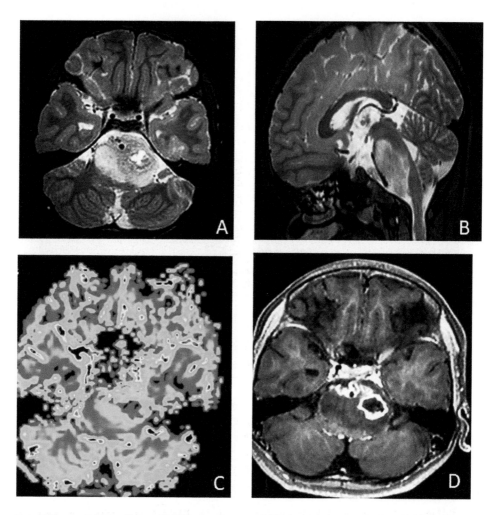

Figure 8.6 Diffuse midline glioma (DMG): An 8-year-old boy presented with headache and vomiting for 2 months. **(A)** Axial and **(B)** Sagittal T2 images show expansile T2 heterogeneously hyperintense lesion in pons, encasing basilar artery. **(C)** DSC image shows increased perfusion within the lesion. **(D)** Axial PC image shows peripheral ring enhancement with non-enhancing component in its posterior aspect.

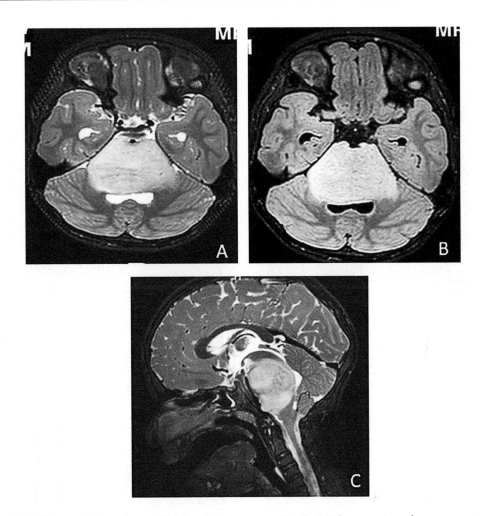

Figure 8.7 Diffuse midline glioma (DMG) – Another case: **(A–C)** DMG are assigned as a separate category of astrocytic tumors in the WHO-2016 classification.

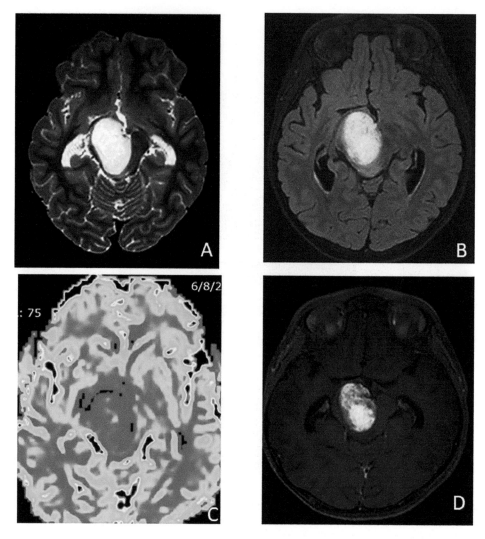

Figure 8.8 Pilocytic astrocytoma (PA): A 10-year-old male child presented with headache, vomiting and decreased vision in both eyes since 3 months. **(A)** Axial T2 and **(B)** FLAIR images show T2 hyperintense lesion in right thalamopeduncular region without showing suppression on FLAIR images. **(C)** DSC perfusion image shows no significant elevated perfusion within the lesion. **(D)** Axial PC image shows intense enhancement.

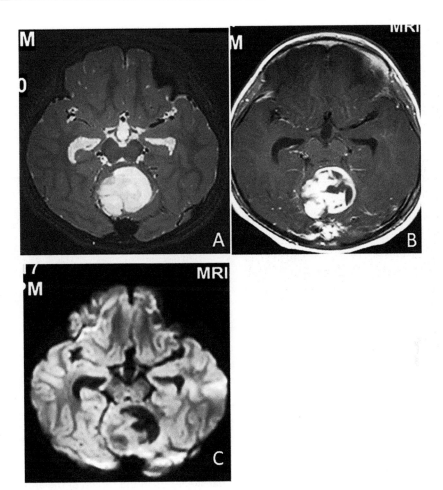

Figure 8.9 Pilocytic astrocytoma (PA) – continued (Another case): **(A)** PAs are usually well marginated, bright on T2-w image, **(B)** Show intense contrast enhancement and have a cyst with mural nodule morphology. **(C)** The DWI does not show diffusion restriction helping to differentiate PA from medulloblastoma, another common posterior fossa tumor in children.

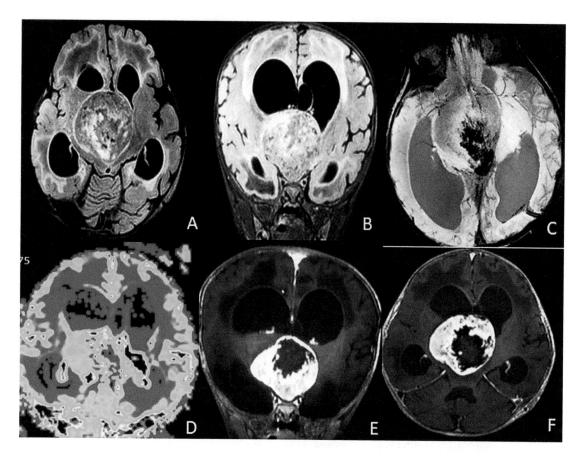

Figure 8.10 Pilomyxoid astrocytoma (PMA): A 4-year-old boy presented with vomiting since 1 month. (A) Axial and (B) Cor FLAIR image showed large expansile lesion in the region of the anterior commissure, suprasellar and hypothalamic region. (C) Axial SWI image shows multiple areas of blooming within the lesion. (D) DSC perfusion study shows increased perfusion within the lesion. (E) Axial and (F) Cor PC images showed intense enhancement with non-enhancing cystic components within. Tumor in the location of the anterior commissure in less than 4 years child with high grade features are commonly pilomyxoid astrocytoma.

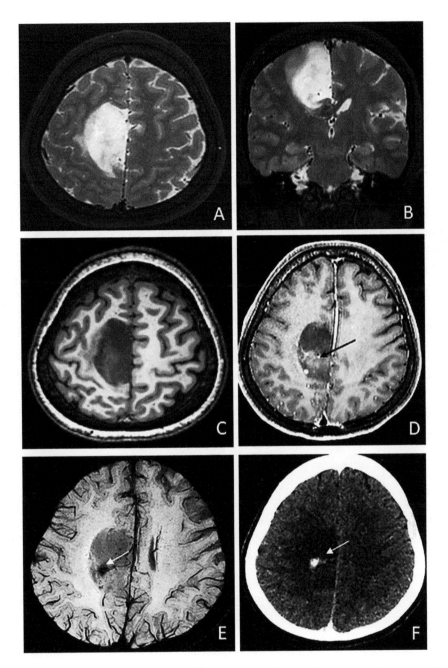

Figure 8.11 Oligodendroglioma: A 55-year-old male complaining of headache since 4 months and one episode of seizure 10 days back. **(A, B)** T2w and **(C, D)** T1PG image shows an intra-axial cortical-based lesion in right medial, superior frontal lobe, causing expansion of the same and shows mild heterogeneous enhancement within central and posterior aspect of the lesion (black arrow). **(E, F)** On SWI, an internal foci of blooming is seen corresponding to calcifications in NCCT image (white arrow). Cortical-based lesion with gyral expansion are imaging features, highly suggestive of oligodendroglioma.

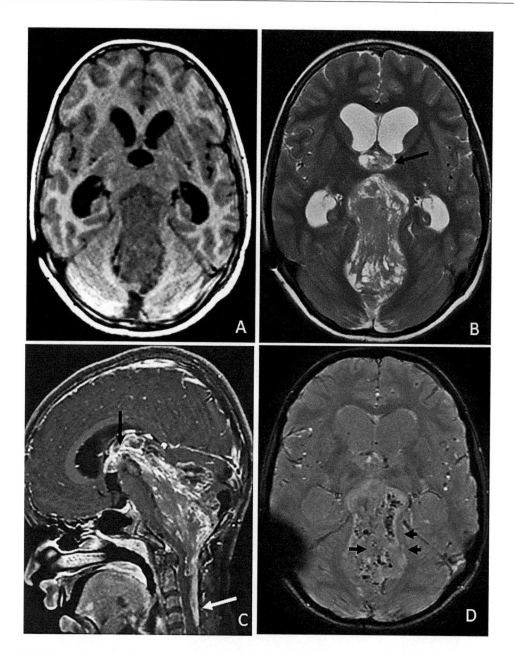

Figure 8.12 Ependymoma: A 14-year-old boy presented with headache, vomiting and blurring of vision. **(A)** Axial T1 and **(B)** T2-w images show heterogeneous intraventricular mass within the fourth ventricle, extending into the third ventricle (black long arrows) through the aqueduct. Note the dilated temporal horns, suggestive of obstructive hydrocephalus. **(C)** Sagittal T1-w post-gadolinium image show, moderate enhancement. Note the extension of the mass through foramen of Magendie into posterior spinal subarachnoid space (white long arrow). **(D)** Axial SWI image shows multiple punctate dark signals, which could be hemorrhages or calcifications.

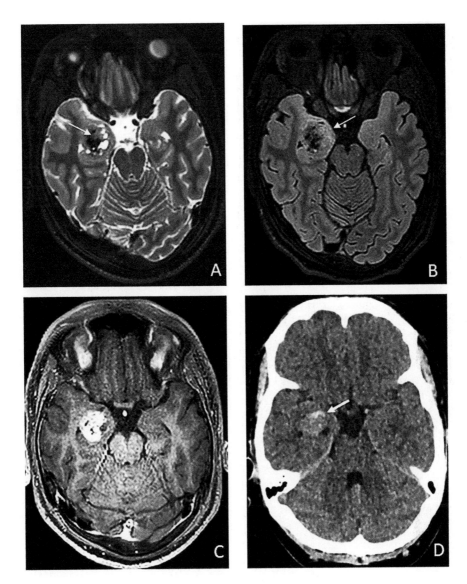

Figure 8.13 Ganglioglioma: A 24-year-old male presented with seizures since 6 years. **(A)** Axial T2, **(B)** FLAIR, and **(C)** T1 PG images show intra-axial lesion involving right medial temporal lobe and hippocampus (thin white arrow) showing heterogeneous enhancement on post-contrast study. **(D)** Axial NCCT image shows internal foci of calcification in its anterior aspect. These imaging features and location are classical of ganglioglioma.

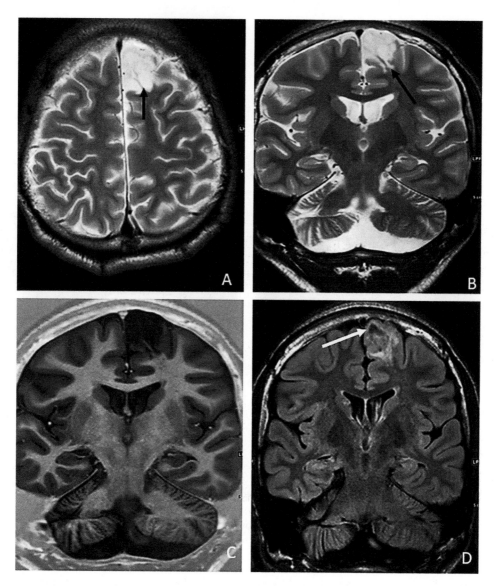

Figure 8.14 Dysembryoplastic neuroepithelial tumor (DNET): A 24-year-old male presented with recurrent seizures. **(A)** Axial and **(B)** coronal T2-w images show cortical-based bubbly, bright lesion involving left frontal lobe (black arrows). **(C)** It is dark in T1-w image. **(D)** Coronal FLAIR image shows suppression in few areas, suggesting cystic areas within the lesion (white arrow).

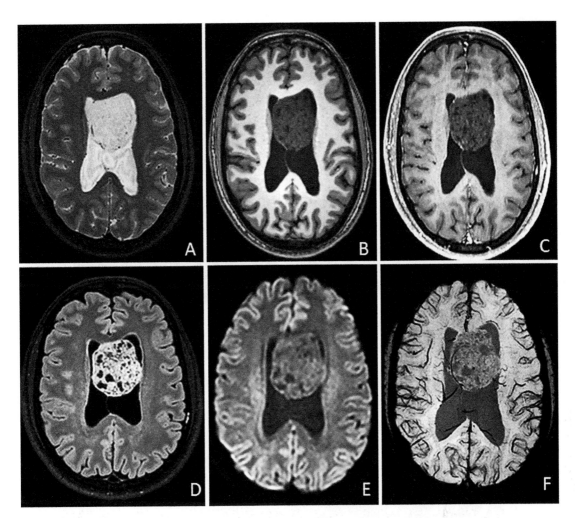

Figure 8.15 Central neurocytoma: A 36-year-old female presented with headache since 3 months and difficulty in walking and maintaining balance for 1 month. **(A)** Axial T2-w and **(D)** FLAIR images show T2 hyperintense lesion with internal cystic areas showing suppression on FLAIR images. The mass is attached to septum pellucidum. **(B, C)** Axial T1-w image shows hypointense lesion without significant enhancement on post-contrast study. **(E)** Axial DWI shows no restricted diffusion and **(F)** SWI shows no areas of blooming within the lesion.

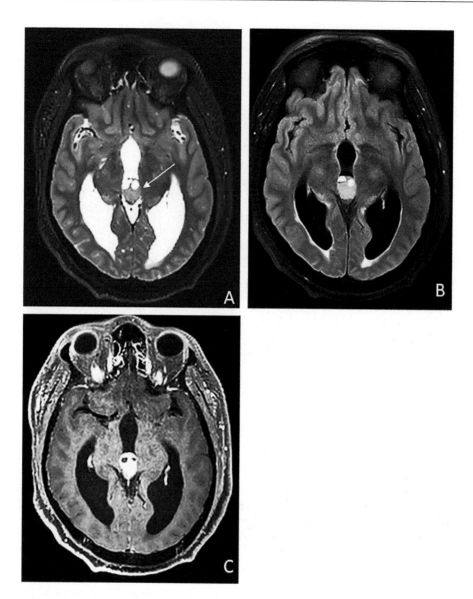

Figure 8.16 Pineocytoma: A 40-year-old female presented with complaints of headache and visual blurring since 4 months. **(A)** Axial T2-w, **(B)** FLAIR, and **(C)** T1-w post-contrast images show ovoid lesion centred in pineal region (white arrow), showing homogeneous enhancement with internal non-enhancing cystic areas. Lesion is causing dilatation of bilateral lateral and third ventricles. The location, age and benign morphology are features of pineocytoma.

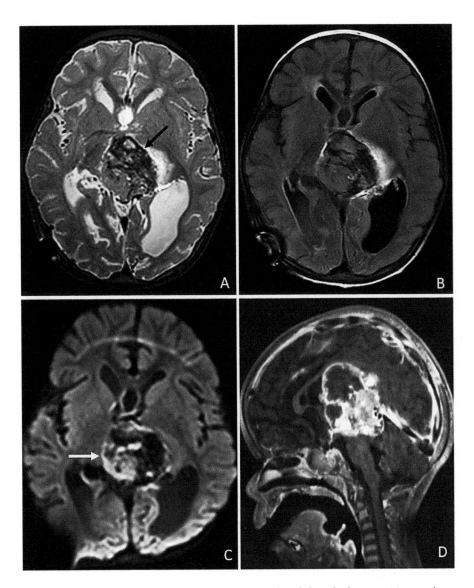

Figure 8.17 Pinealoblastoma: An 8-year-old boy presented with headache, vomiting and gaze palsy.
(A) Axial T2 and **(B)** FLAIR images show a large heterogeneous mass in the region of posterior third ventricle and pineal gland. Anterior aspect of the mass shows multiple dark areas (black arrow), which could represent calcification or hemorrhages. **(C)** Bright appearance is seen in the DWI (white arrow), suggestive of diffusion restriction, indicating increased cellularity. **(D)** Post-contrast sagittal image shows moderate to intense heterogeneous enhancement.

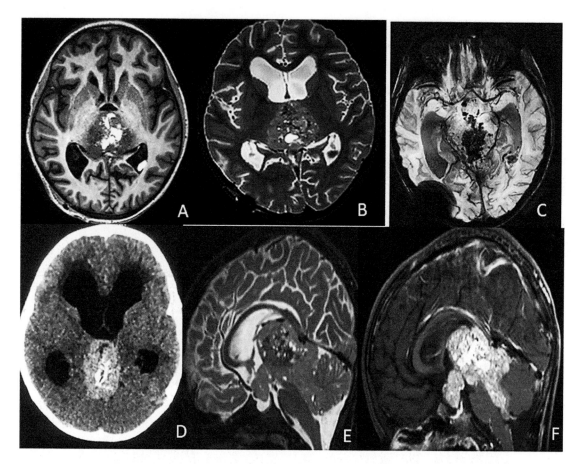

Figure 8.18 Pineal and suprasellar germinoma: A 12-year-old boy presented with headache and vomiting for 1 month. **(A)** Axial T1, **(B)** T2, and **(E)** Saggital T2 images show heterogeneously iso to hyperintense lesion in the pineal and suprasellar region showing central calcification on **(C)** SWI images in the pineal region. **(D)** Axial NCCT image shows central calcification within the tumor. **(F)** Saggital T1 PC image shows intense enhancement within the lesions. Central calcification is commonly associated with pineal germinoma while peripheral calcification is seen in pinealoblastoma.

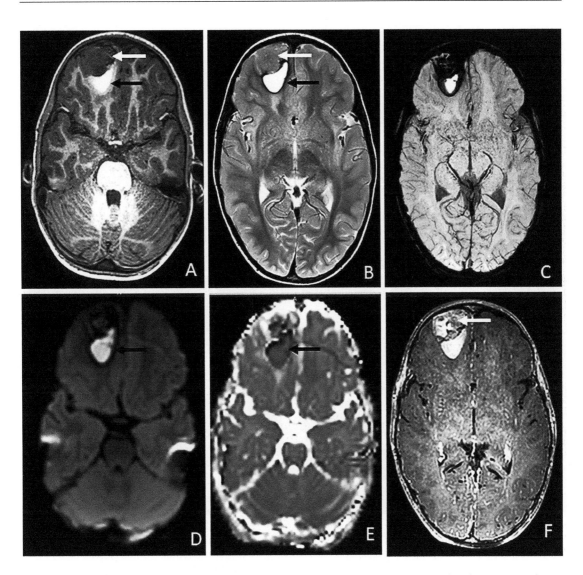

Figure 8.19 Atypical teratoid rhabdoid tumor: A 3-year-old male child presented with two episodes of seizures. **(A)** Axial T1 and **(B)** T2-w images show well-defined, solid, intra-parenchymal lesion in the right frontal lobe (white arrows). Posterior to the lesion, there is a focal area of T1 and T2 hyperintense signal suggestive of hemorrhage (black arrows). **(C)** Axial SWI shows blooming in the lesion, suggestive of hemorrhage. **(D)** Axial DWI trace and **(E)** ADC map shows the hemorrhage to be hyperintense and hypointense respectively, suggestive of diffusion restriction. **(F)** Post gadolinium T1-w image shows heterogeneous enhancement of the tumor.

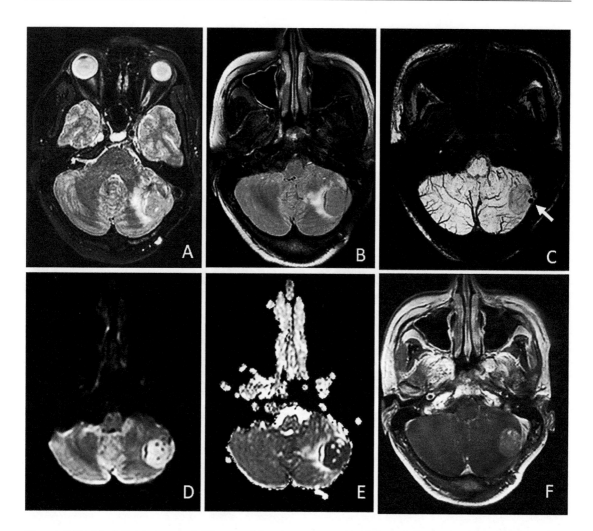

Figure 8.20 Medulloblastoma: A 27-year-old male presented with headache and vomiting. **(A)** Axial T2-w and **(B)** FLAIR images show a well-defined rounded, intra-parenchymal, nodular lesion in the left cerebellar hemisphere with mild perilesional edema. **(C)** Axial SWI shows a single focus of microhemorrhage, seen as a hypointense dot (white arrow). **(D)** Axial DWI trace and **(E)** ADC map shows hyperintense and hypointense appearance respectively, suggestive of diffusion restriction. **(F)** Post gadolinium T1-w image shows mild homogeneous solid enhancement.

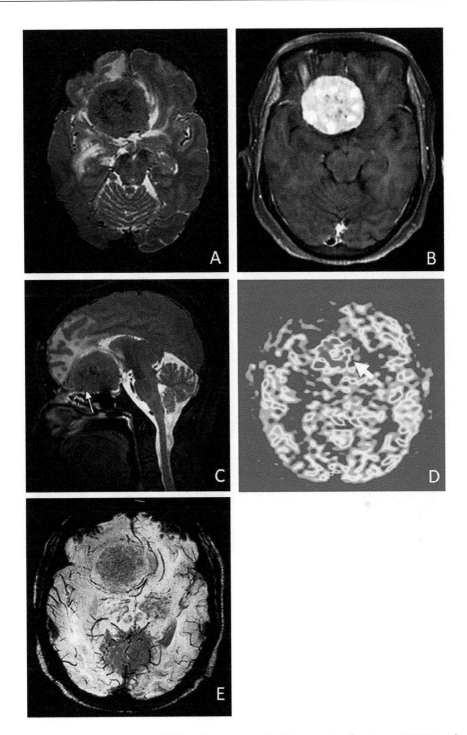

Figure 8.21 Meningioma: A 56-year-old female presented with headache for 1 year. (A) T2 and
(B, C) T1PGw images show broad-based extra-axial lesion attached to the cribriform plate (white
arrow), showing intense heterogeneous enhancement on post-contrast study. (E) On SWI, no internal
foci of blooming is seen. (D) On ASL, lesion shows hyper-perfusion (thick white arrow).

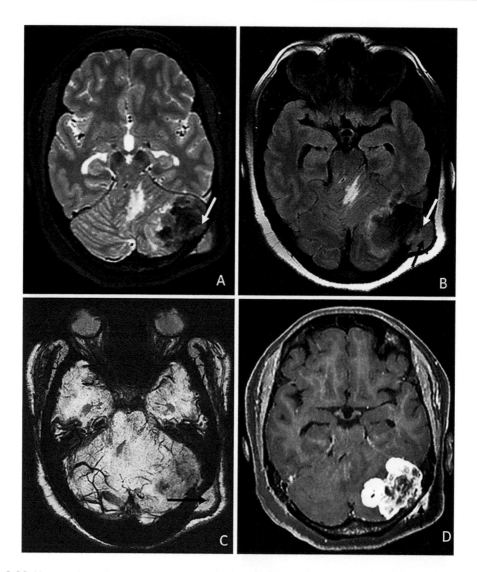

Figure 8.22 Hemangiopericytoma: A 35-year-old female presented with occipital headache since 1 year. **(A)** Axial T2-w and **(B)** FLAIR images show heterogeneous, predominantly hypointense lesion in the left side of the posterior fossa, with mass effect over the cerebellum and fourth ventricle, and perilesional edema. It is seen eroding the occipital bone, with a small soft tissue component in the scalp. **(C)** Axial SWI shows no significant blooming to suggest hemorrhage or calcification. **(D)** Axial T1-w post-gadolinium image shows heterogeneous intense enhancement. Note the bone erosion (white arrows) and extra-cranial scalp component (black arrows).

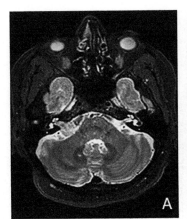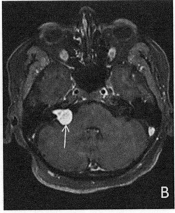

Figure 8.23 Right acoustic schwannoma: **(A, B)** Brightly enhancing mass lesion in the right internal acoustic canal expanding into the cerebellopontine angle cistern with characteristic ice cream cone appearance.

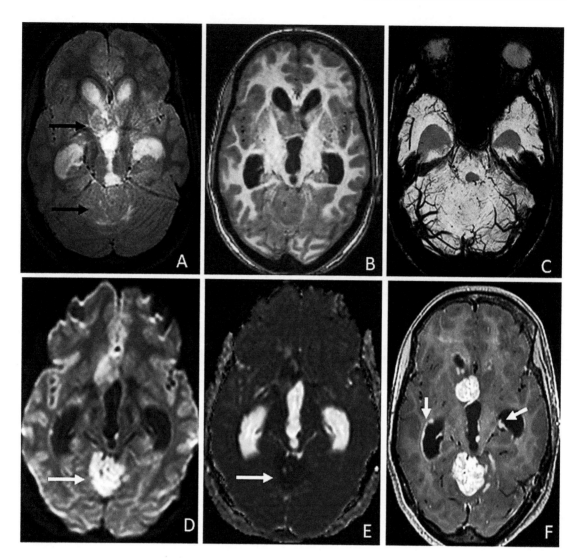

Figure 8.24 Lymphoma: A 43-year-old female presented with headache and giddiness for 6 months. **(A)** Axial T2 and **(B)** T1 images show two rounded solid lesions (black arrows). **(C)** Axial SWI shows no dark areas to suggest hemorrhage or calcifications. **(D, E)** Bright appearance on DWI and dark appearance in ADC (white long arrows) is indicative of diffusion restriction suggesting hypercellularity. **(F)** Note other multiple subependymal enhancing nodules (white arrows).

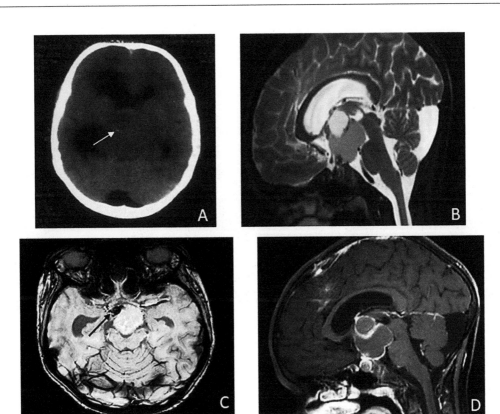

Figure 8.25 Craniopharyngioma: A 10-year-old male child presented with headache, vomiting and gradual progressive loss of vision in both eyes. **(A)** Axial NCCT scan shows relatively well defined solid-cystic lesion with peripheral calcification in suprasellar region (white arrow). **(C)** Axial SWI image shows peripheral blooming corresponding to areas of calcification on NCCT scan (black arrow). The lesion shows heterogenous hyperintensity on **(B)** sagittal T2-w images with peripheral enhancement on post-contrast study **(D)**.

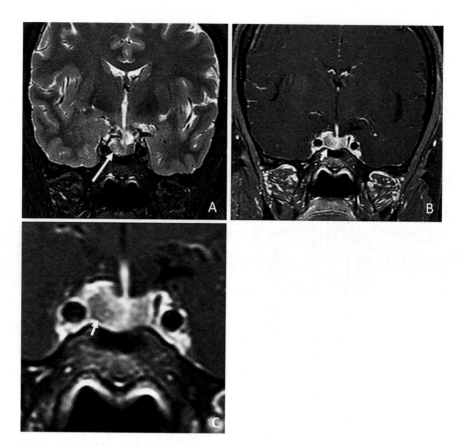

Figure 8.26 Pituitary microadenoma: A 29-year-old female presented with irregular menstrual cycles for 6 months. **(A)** Coronal T2-w image at the level of sella shows focally enlarged pituitary gland, in the right side, which also appears hyperintense compared with rest of the pituitary gland (white long arrow). **(B, C)** Post gadolinium administration, the right side of the pituitary gland shows a rounded, sub-centimetric, hypoenhancing lesion in T1-w images, suggestive of pituitary microadenoma (short white arrow).

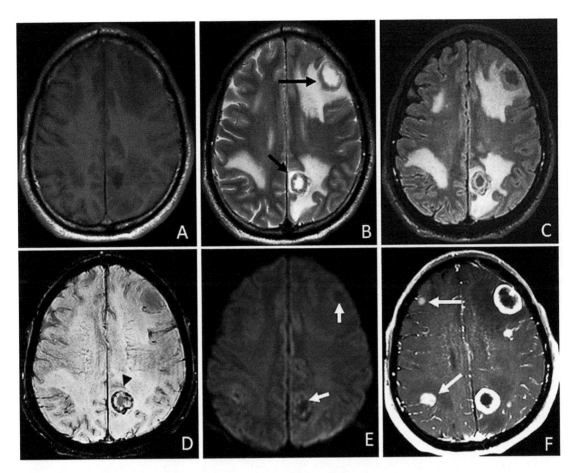

Figure 8.27 Metastasis: A 49-year-old man presented with loss of weight and altered sensorium.
(A) Axial T1, (B) T2, and (C) FLAIR images show multiple ring lesions with perilesional edema (black arrows). (D) Few of the ring lesions show dark areas in SW, suggestive of hemorrhages (black arrowhead). (E) The rims appear brighter in DWI, suggestive of diffusion restriction (short white arrows). (F) These lesions show thick ring enhancement in T1 post-contrast image. Note that multiple other nodular enhancing lesions (long white arrows) are seen. Lung, kidney, breast, GIT and melanoma are five primary tumors that account for more than 80% metastases.

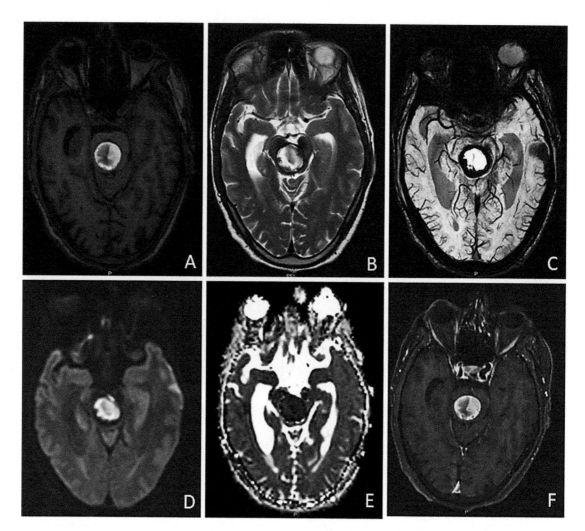

Figure 8.28 Melanocytoma: A 39-year-old adult presented with slowly progressive asymmetric weakness of all four limbs with slurring of speech. **(A)** Axial T1-w and **(B)** T2-w images show a well-defined, rounded, predominantly hyperintense lesion in the pons with hypointense areas, and no perilesional edema. **(C)** Axial SWI image shows hemorrhage in the periphery of the mass. **(D)** DWI trace and **(E)** ADC map shows hyperintense and hypointense appearance respectively, suggestive of diffusion restriction. **(F)** Axial T1-w post-gadolinium image show same appearance as that of the pre-contrast image. T1-w hyperintense appearance is characteristic of melanoma.

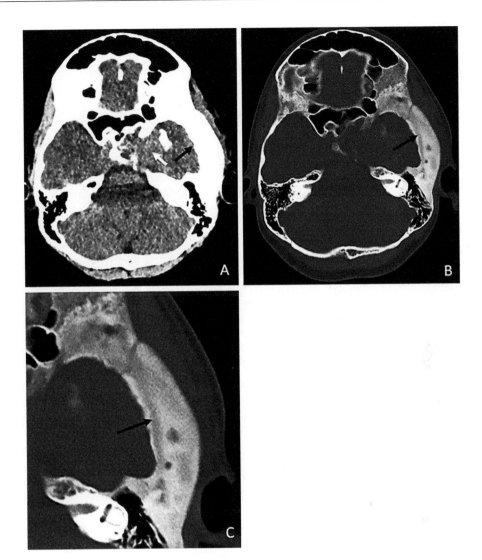

Figure 8.29 Fibrous dysplasia: A 22-year-old male presented with bony swelling on the left side of the face. **(A–C)** Axial NCCT image (brain window) shows thickening of the left temporal bone (black arrow). Axial images in bone window shows thickening of squamous part of left temporal bone with marrow showing 'ground-glass' appearance with indistinct inner and outer table of skull. Note is also made of incidental left parasellar mass lesion (white arrow).

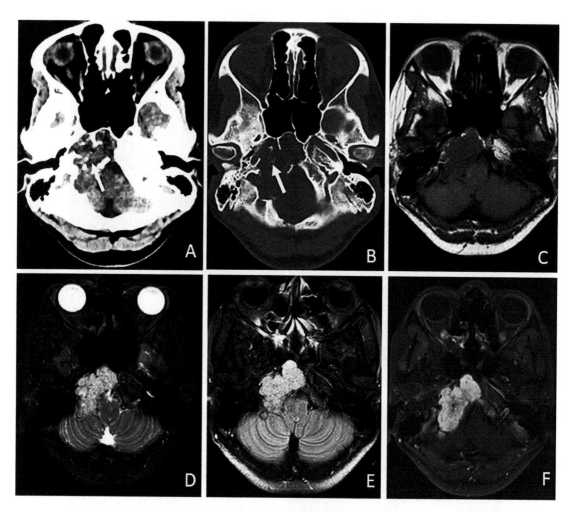

Figure 8.30 Chondromyxoid fibroma of skull base: A 20-year-old female presented neck pain and difficulty in swallowing for the last 3 months. **(A)** Axial NCCT image of the brain in brain and **(B)** bone window settings show well-defined, expansile, lytic lesion in the right side of the skull base involving petrous and occipital bones (white arrows). **(C)** Axial T1-w image shows hypointense appearance of the lesion. **(D)** Axial T2-w and **(E)** FLAIR images show lobulated hyperintense appearance. **(F)** T1-w post-gadolinium image shows homogeneous enhancement.

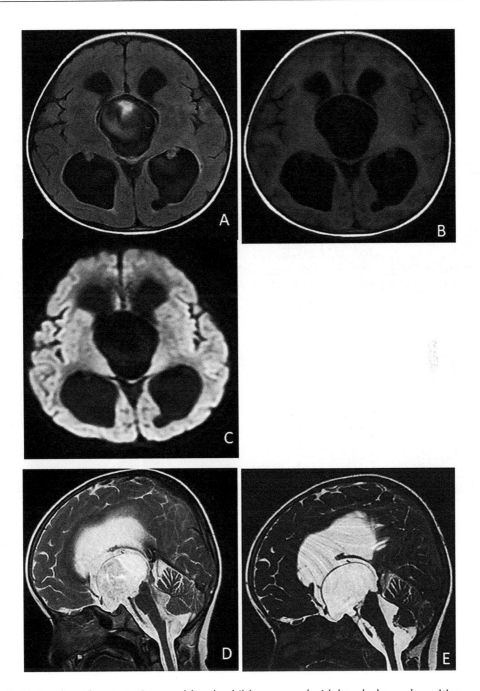

Figure 8.31 Arachnoid cyst: A 12-year-old male child presented with headache and vomiting for 3 months. **(A)** Axial FLAIR, **(B)** T1-w, **(D)** Sagittal T2-w images show CSF intensity lesion in suprasellar region displacing the third ventricle superiorly with hydrocephalus. **(C)** Axial DWI image shows no restricted diffusion. **(E)** Sagittal DRIVE image clearly shows thin membranous wall of the arachnoid cyst.

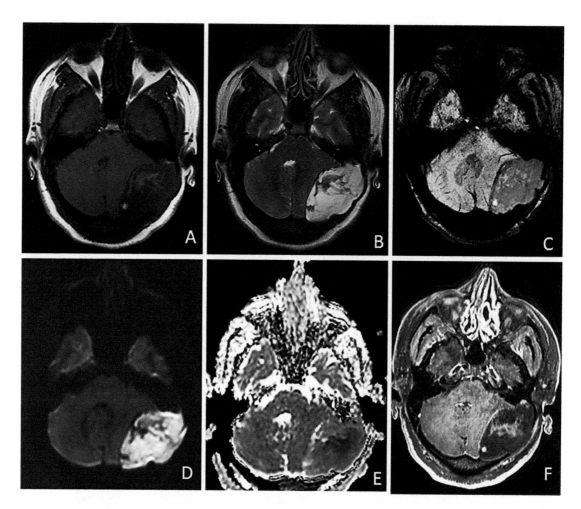

Figure 8.32 Intradiploic epidermoid cyst: A middle-aged man presented with history of headache. **(A)** Axial T1 and **(B)** T2-w images of the brain show expansile lytic lesion of left side of the occipital bone. It is predominantly hypointense in T1 and hyperintense in T2-w images, with few T1 hyperintense and T2 hypointense areas. **(C)** Axial SWI shows no hemorrhage or calcification. **(D)** Axial DWI trace and **(E)** ADC map shows hyperintense and hypointense appearance respectively, suggestive of diffusion restriction. **(F)** Axial T1-w post-gadolinium image shows no enhancement.

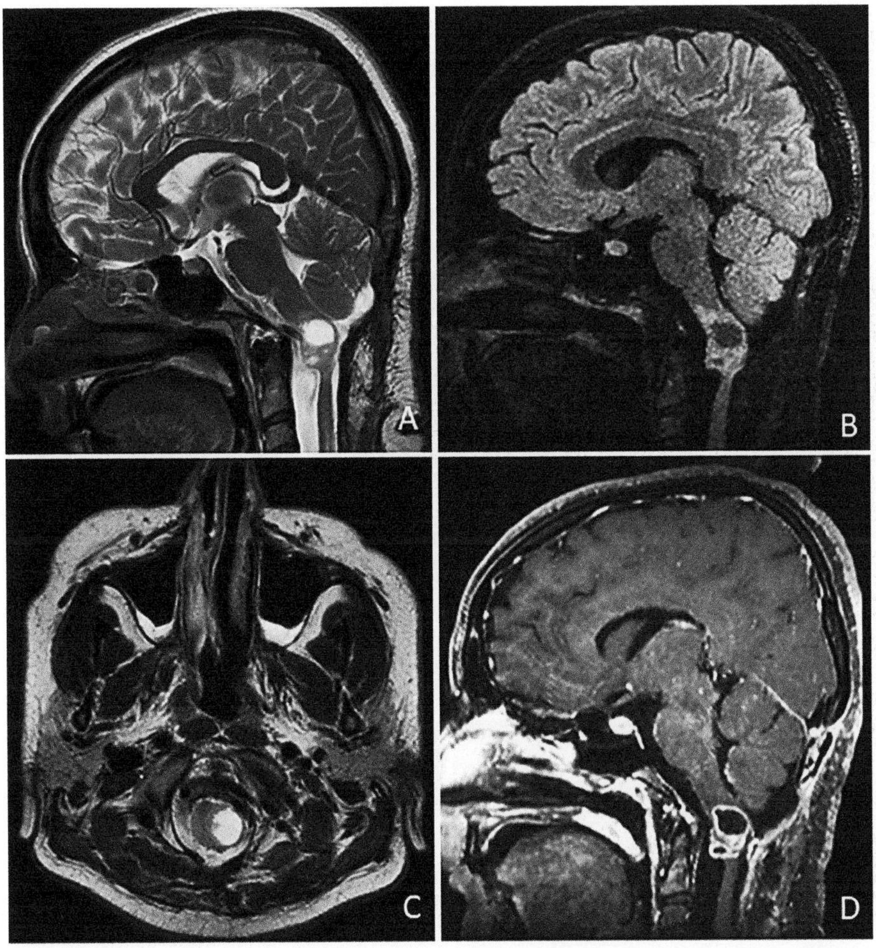

Figure 8.33 Ganglioglioma: A 30-year-old female presented with headache with gradual progressive weakness involving all four limbs for 3 months. **(A)** Sagittal T2, **(B)** FLAIR and **(C)** Axial T2-w images show relatively well-defined solid cystic lesion in cervicomedullary junction showing suppression of cystic part on FLAIR image. **(D)** Sagittal T1-w post-contrast image shows irregular peripheral enhancement.

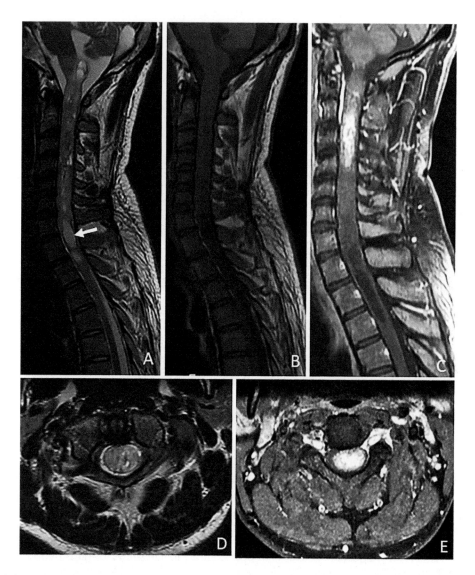

Figure 8.34 Astrocytoma: A 15-year-old male presented with complaints of progressive paraparesis and numbness in both lower limbs for 1 year. **(A)** Sagittal and **(D)** axial T2-w images show well-defined solid cystic intramedullary lesion extending from D3 to D10 level with heterogeneously hyperintense solid component and perilesional edema. **(B)** Sagittal T1-w image shows that the solid component is isointense. **(C)** Sagittal and **(E)** axial T1-w post-contrast images show intense enhancement of the solid component and peripheral rim enhancement of the cystic component. Note is made of syrinx extending from C6 to D2 level (white arrow).

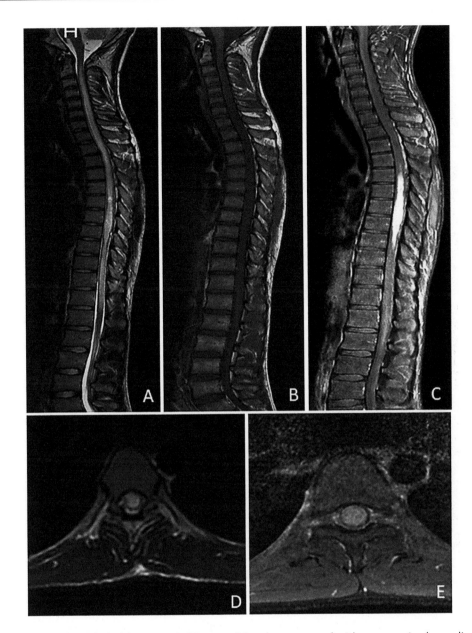

Figure 8.35 Spinal cord glioblastoma: A 23-year-old male presented with progressive lower limb weakness and sensory loss. **(A)** Sagittal and **(D)** axial T2-w images show long segment hyperintense lesion in cervicodorsal region with cord expansion. **(B)** Sagittal T1-w image shows hypointense signal. **(C)** Sagittal and **(E)** axial T1-w post-contrast images show long segment of intense enhancement in the mid-dorsal cord.

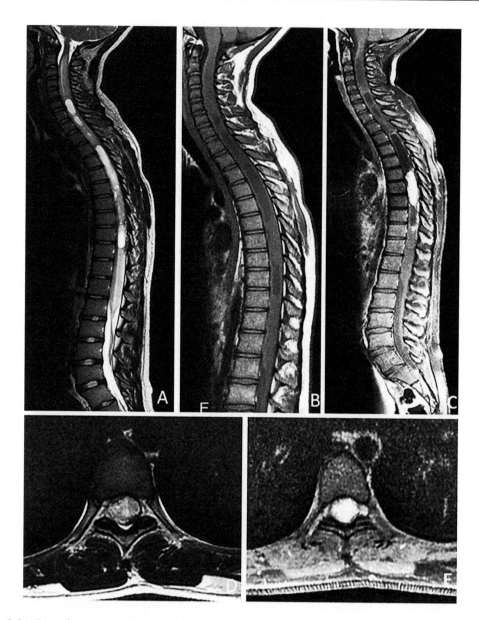

Figure 8.36 Ependymoma: A 33-year-old male presented with complaints of progressive weakness involving all four limbs. **(A)** Sagittal and **(D)** axial T2-w images show long segment mixed solid-cystic central intramedullary lesion extending from cervicomedullary junction to D3 vertebral level. **(B)** Sagittal T1-w image shows that the lesion is hypointense. Holocord syrinx is seen in T2-w image. **(C, E)** Sagittal and axial T1-w post-contrast images show heterogeneous enhancement of the solid component and peripheral enhancement of the cystic component.

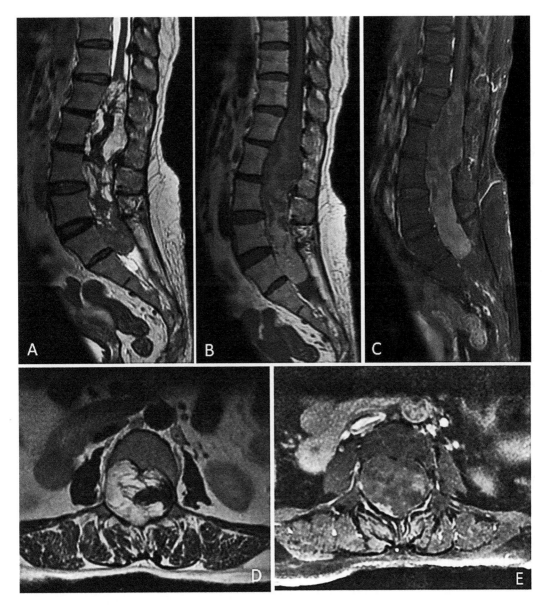

Figure 8.37 Myxopapillary ependymoma: A 52-year-old female presented with complaints of low backache and bilateral lower limb weakness for 1 year. **(A)** Sagittal and **(D)** axial T2-w images show a large lobulated hyperintense mass filling the lumbosacral thecal sac causing scalloping and remodeling of posterior lumbar vertebral bodies. **(B)** Saggital T1 image shows heterogeneously hypointense lesion. **(C)** Saggital T1+C and **(E)** axial T1+C image demonstrates heterogeneous enhancement within the lesion.

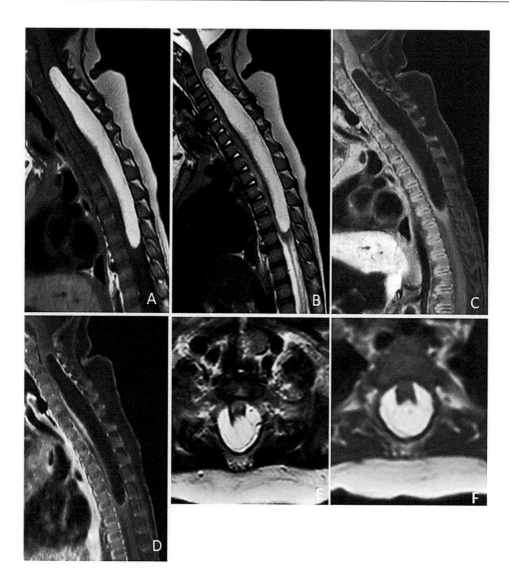

Figure 8.38 Lipoma: A 6-year-old female presented with complaints of swelling in upper back and weakness involving all four limbs. **(A)** Sagittal T1, **(B)** T2, **(F)** axial T1 and **(E)** T2-w images show well-defined hyperintense intramedullary/surface lesion in dorsal aspect of the cervicodorsal cord without any enhancement in **(D)** sagittal T1 post-contrast image. **(C)** Note that lesion is completely suppressed in T1 fat-saturated image, indicating the fat component of the lesion.

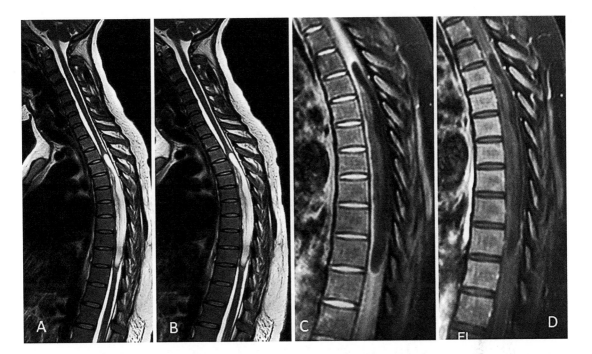

Figure 8.39 Angiolipoma: A 28-year-old female presented with bilateral lower limb paraparesis for 6 months. **(A, B)** Sagittal T2-w images show heterogeneous hyperintense intradural subpial lesion extending from D3-D11 levels causing obliteration of cord-CSF interface both anteriorly and posteriorly. The T2-w images show hyperintense posterior component and hypointense anterior component. **(C)** Sagittal T1-w fat-saturated image shows suppression of posterior hyperintense fat component of the tumor. **(D)** Sagittal T1-w post-contrast image shows mild peripheral enhancement of anterior component, indicating angiomatous component of the tumor.

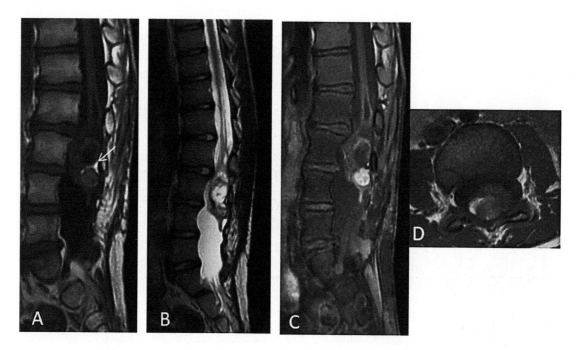

Figure 8.40 Conus dermoid: A 24-year-old male presented with bladder and bowel incontinence for 1 year. **(A)** Sagittal T1 image shows heterogeneous expansile lesion in the region of the conus with hyperintense fat within (white arrow). **(B)** Sagittal T2 image shows lesion is heterogeneously hyperintense and **(C)** sagittal PC image shows minimal enhancement of the most part of the lesion with intense enhancement of the posterior aspect. **(D)** Axial T1 image shows peripheral T1 hyperintensity in the region of the fat. Conus is the common location of the dermoid in the spine.

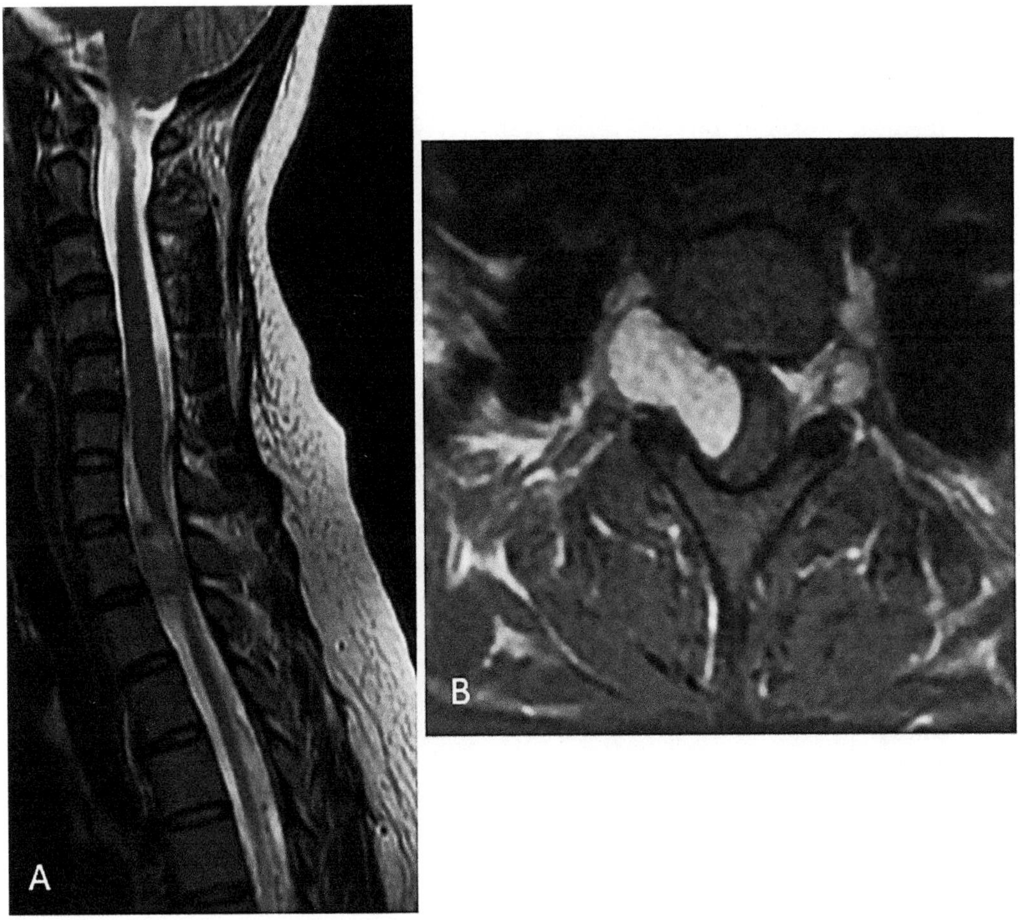

Figure 8.41 Schwannoma: A 30-year-old female presented with unsteady gait for 1 year. **(A)** Sagittal T2-w image shows well-defined heterogeneously iso to hyperintense intradural extramedullary lesion at D1 level, anterior to the cord. **(B)** Axial T1-w post-contrast image shows that the lesion is extending into the neural foramen, having typical dumbbell shape, with homogeneous solid enhancement of the lesion.

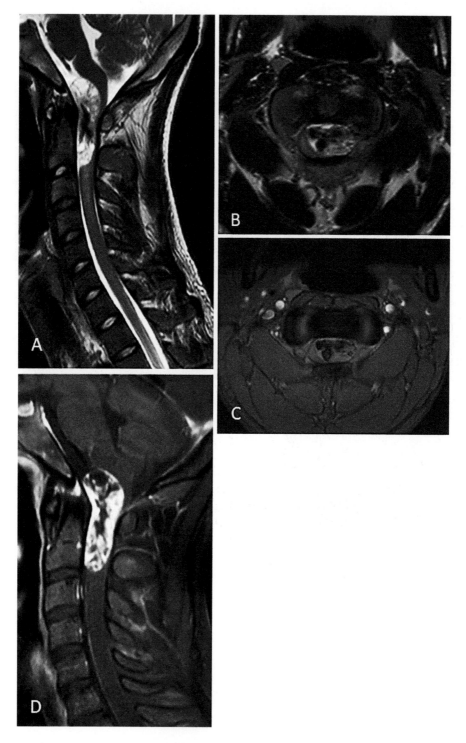

Figure 8.42 Schwannoma – continued: A 24-year-old male presented with progressive spastic weakness in left upper limb followed by progressive weakness of all four limbs. **(A)** Sagittal and **(B)** axial T2-w images show well-defined heterogeneously hyperintense intradural extramedullary lesion in high cervical region extending into neural foramen. Lesion is causing displacement and compression of cervical spinal cord. **(C)** Axial GRE image shows internal areas of blooming within the lesion. **(D)** Sagittal T1-w post-contrast image shows intense heterogeneous enhancement.

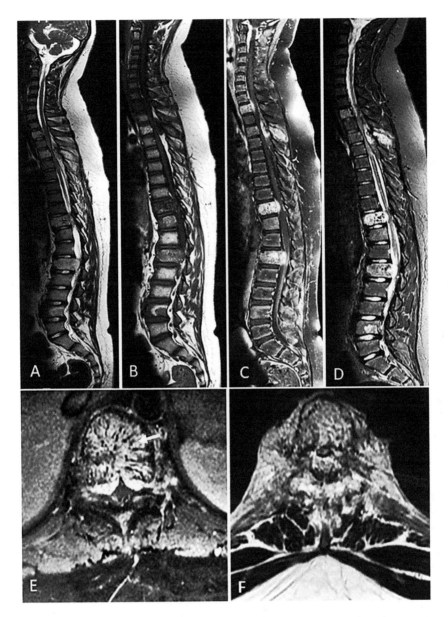

Figure 8.43 Multiple hemangiomas: **(A)** Sagittal and **(E)** axial T2-w images show heterogeneously hyperintense lesion involving multiple dorsal and lumbar vertebral bodies with extra-osseous component in bilateral paravertebral regions, also extending into epidural spaces causing displacement and compression of spinal cord with cord signal changes. **(B)** The involved vertebrae appear hypointense on T1. **(D)** Sagittal STIR image shows incomplete suppression of signal within the lesions, indicating active vascular component of the lesion. Axial images show polka-dot appearance which is characteristic of hemangioma (white arrow). **(C)** Sagittal and **(F)** axial T1-w post-contrast images show heterogeneous enhancement.

Central nervous system infections

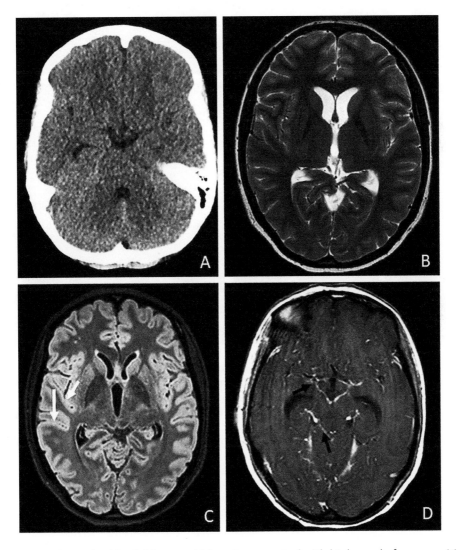

9

Figure 9.1 Pyogenic meningitis: A 20-year-old female presented with high-grade fever, vomiting, and altered behavior. **(A)** Axial NCCT and **(B)** T2-w images show mildly dilated ventricular system. **(C)** FLAIR image shows hyperintense signals within the sulci, suggestive of exudates (white arrows). **(D)** Axial T1 post-gadolinium image shows linear enhancement in the basal cisterns and in the sulcal spaces (black arrows). Tentorial enhancement is also seen.

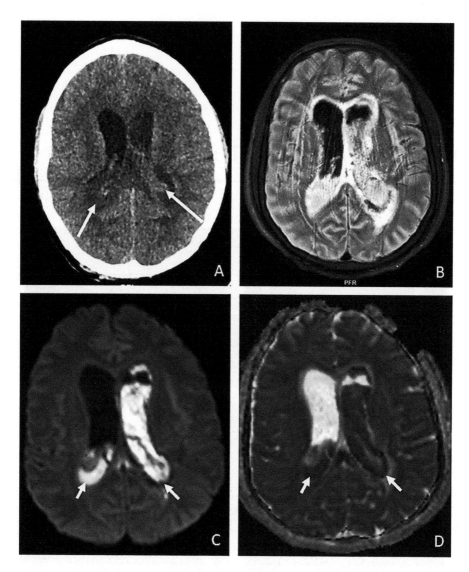

Figure 9.2 Ventriculitis: A 33-year-old man presented with fever and altered sensorium since 2 days, with multiple episodes of seizures. **(A)** Axial NCCT image shows dilated lateral ventricles. Dependent portion of both lateral ventricles show hyperdense pus within (white long arrows). **(B)** Axial FLAIR image shows intraventricular hyperintense signal, dilated ventricles with periventricular seepage of CSF. **(C)** Diffusion trace images show intraventricular hyperintense signal with corresponding regions in **(D)** ADC map showing low values (white short arrows), suggestive of diffusion restriction, consistent with pus.

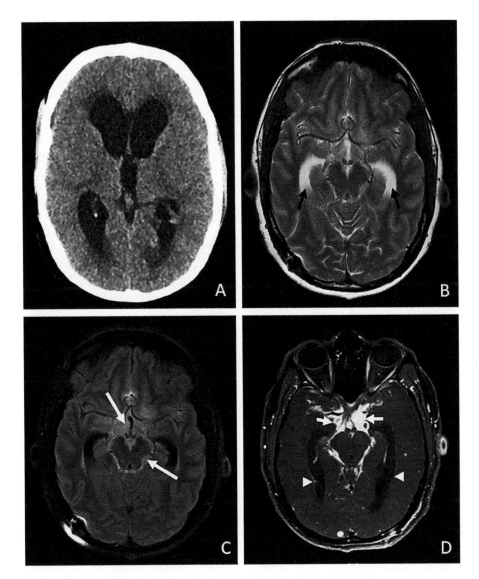

Figure 9.3 Tubercular meningitis: A 27-year-old male presented with seizures. **(A)** Axial NCCT image shows hydrocephalus with periventricular seepage. **(B)** Axial T2-w image shows dilated temporal horns of lateral ventricles (black arrows). **(C)** Axial FLAIR image shows hyperintense signals in basal cisterns suggestive of exudates (white long arrows). **(D)** Axial T1 post-gadolinium image shows thick enhancement in the basal cisterns and along the optic nerves and chiasm (white short arrows). Thin ependymal enhancement is also seen along the ependymal lining of both lateral ventricles (white arrowheads).

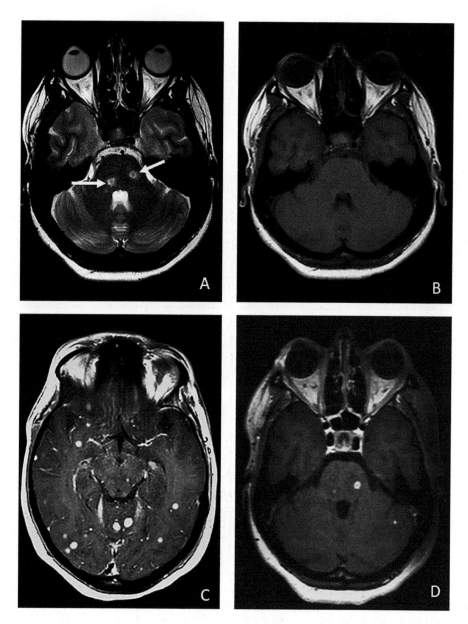

Figure 9.4 Tuberculoma: A 33-year-old female presented with 2 months of low-grade fever and sudden onset of altered sensorium. **(A)** T2-w axial image shows multiple hypointense nodular lesions with a rim of hyperintense perilesional edema (white arrow). The lesions are isointense in **(B)** axial T1-w image. **(C, D)** Axial T1-w post-gadolinium images show multiple small ring and solid nodular enhancing lesions distributed throughout brain parenchyma.

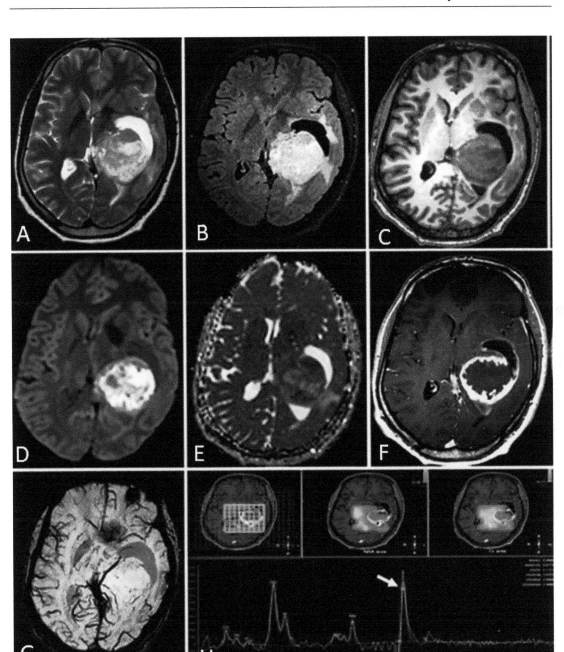

Figure 9.5 Giant tuberculoma: A 31-year-old female presented with headache and vomiting since 3 months. **(A–C)** Axial T2, FLAIR, and T1-w images show T2 heterogeneous hyperintense and T1 hypointense lesion adjacent to atrium of left lateral ventricle. **(D, E)** Axial DWI and ADC images show restricted diffusion within the lesion and **(G)** SWI image shows no blooming. **(F)** Axial T1-w post-contrast image show smooth enhancement of the outer wall with inner irregular margin, extending along atrium of left lateral ventricle. **(H)** MRS shows reduced NAA and increased lipid-lactate peak (white arrow).

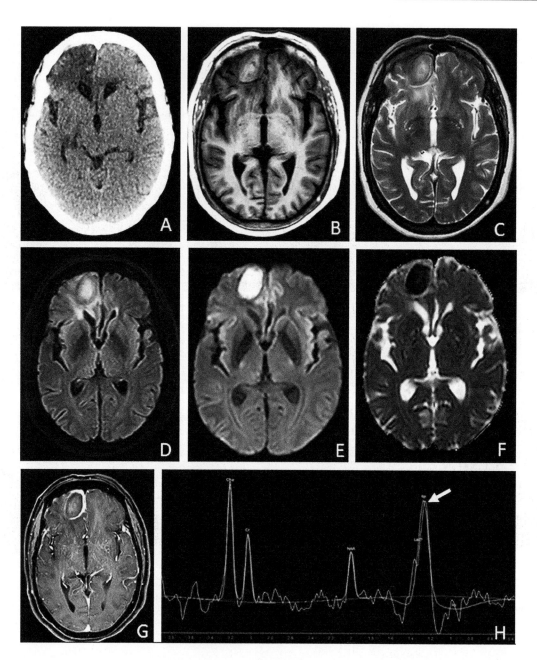

Figure 9.6 Fungal abscess: A 51-year-old male presented with incoherent talking and altered behavior for the past 2 days. **(A)** Axial NCCT image shows right frontal region hypodensity. **(B, C)** Axial T1 and T2-w images show well-defined ovoid T1 iso to hyperintense and T2 iso to hypointense lesion with perilesional edema. **(D)** It appears hyperintense in the center and hypointense in the periphery in FLAIR image. **(E)** Diffusion trace image shows hyperintense appearance, with corresponding areas in **(F)** ADC map showing low values, suggestive of diffusion restriction. **(G)** Axial T1 post-gadolinium image shows thick peripheral ring enhancement. **(H)** MR spectroscopy shows a large lactate peak at 1.3 ppm (white arrow), suggestive of anaerobic metabolism in the region, which is consistent with abscess.

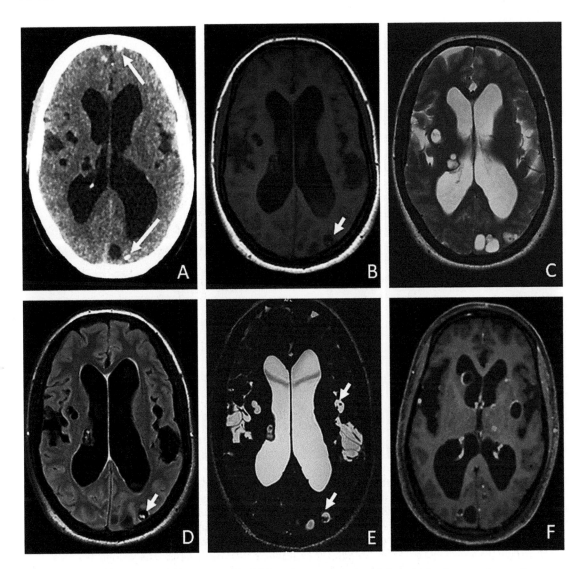

Figure 9.7 Neurocysticercosis: A 38-year-old female presented with headache for past 6 months and blurring of vision. **(A)** Axial NCCT image shows multiple rounded hypodense lesions with density similar to CSF. No perilesional edema is seen. Few nodular calcifications are also seen (white long arrows). **(B, C)** Axial T1-w and T2-w images show multiple rounded cystic lesions with CSF like intensity. Few nodular areas are seen within the cysts suggestive of scolex (small white arrows). **(D)** Axial FLAIR image shows complete suppression of cystic content, except for the scolices. **(E)** Axial BTFE image shows the cysts and scolices clearly. **(F)** Axial T1 post-gadolinium image shows few of the lesions showing ring enhancement.

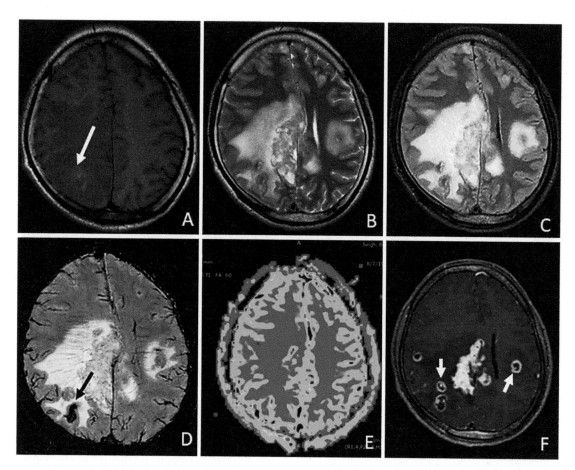

Figure 9.8 Toxoplasmosis: A 22-year-old male with immunocompromised status, presented with headache and vomiting for the past 1 month without any neurological deficits. (B, C) Axial T2 and FLAIR images show multiple heterogeneous lesions with iso to hypointense signal in both posterior frontal and parietal lobes with perilesional edema. (A) Axial T1-w image shows a focus of hyperintense signal suggestive of hemorrhage (white arrow). (D) This is seen as hypointense signal in SWI image (black arrow). (E) Axial DSC perfusion image shows no increased perfusion in the lesions. (F) Axial T1 post-gadolinium image shows confluent solid nodular enhancing lesions and multiple ring-enhancing lesions. Most of the ring enhancing lesions show eccentric enhancing nodule, suggestive of eccentric target sign (white short arrows).

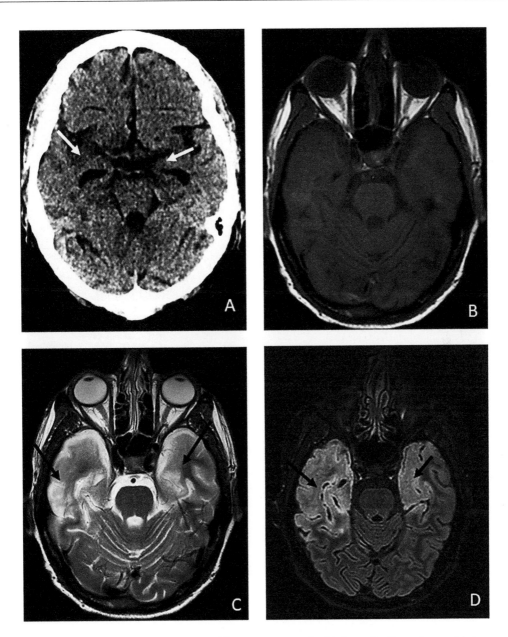

Figure 9.9 Herpes encephalitis: A 34-year-old man presented with fever for 2 weeks, multiple episodes of seizures, and altered sensorium. **(A)** Axial NCCT image shows patchy areas of hypodensities involving both temporal lobes (white arrows). **(B)** Axial T1-w image is unremarkable. **(C, D)** Axial T2-w and FLAIR images show asymmetrical (Rt > Lt) confluent hyperintensities involving both grey and white matter of both temporal lobes (black arrows).

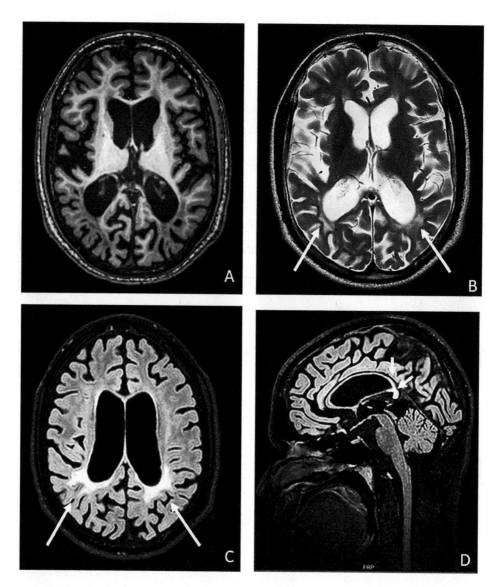

Figure 9.10 Subacute sclerosing panencephalitis: A 24-year-old male presented with slowly progressive cognitive decline over 3 months with acute onset of cortical type of visual loss. **(A)** Axial T1-w image shows diffuse supratentorial brain atrophy with secondary dilatation of ventricles. **(B)** Axial T2-w and **(C)** FLAIR images show confluent, white matter hyperintensities involving parietal deep and periventricular white matter (white long arrows). **(D)** Sagittal FLAIR image of the brain shows hyperintensity involving the posterior body and splenium of corpus callosum (white short arrows). Patient also showed anti-measles IgG antibody positive in CSF.

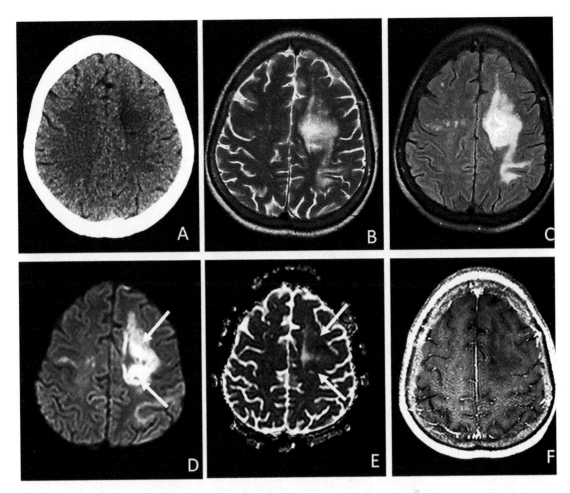

Figure 9.11 Progressive multifocal leukoencephalopathy (PML): A 61-year-old female with history of dermatomyositis and treatment with rituximab, presented with progressive weakness of right upper and lower limb over 2 weeks. (A) Axial NCCT image shows confluent white matter hypodensity involving the left frontal white matter. (B) Axial T2-w and (C) FLAIR images show confluent white matter lesion involving left frontoparietal white matter without significant mass effect. (D) Diffusion-weighted image show peripheral bright signal, and corresponding areas in (E) ADC map shows low values, suggestive of diffusion restriction in the periphery (white arrows). (F) No enhancement is seen in axial T1 post-gadolinium image.

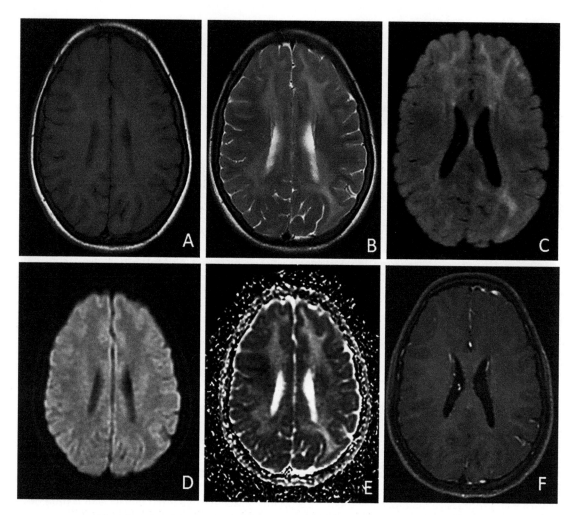

Figure 9.12 Human immunodeficiency virus (HIV) encephalopathy: A 17-year-old girl, with HIV-AIDS and on ART for the last 7 years, developed non-specific neurologic symptoms and mild cognitive decline. **(A)** Axial T1 image appears normal. **(B)** Axial T2 and **(C)** FLAIR images show confluent, symmetrical white matter hyperintensities involving frontal and parietal lobes, predominantly the deep and periventricular white matter. **(D)** Diffusion trace images show no abnormal signals. **(E)** ADC map shows high values suggestive of facilitated diffusion. **(F)** Axial T1 post-gadolinium image shows no enhancement.

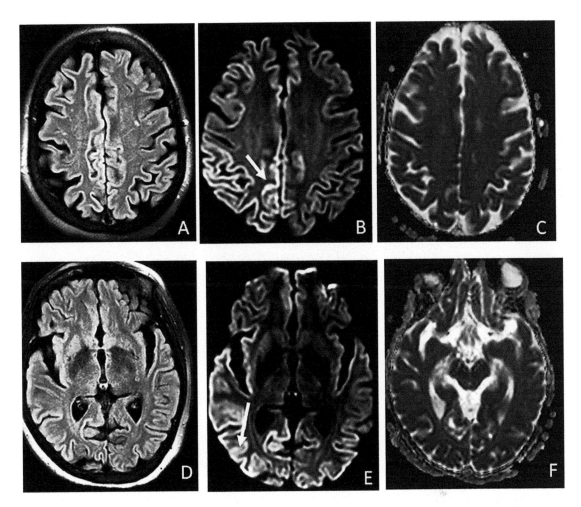

Figure 9.13 Sporadic Creutzfeldt–Jakob disease (CJD): A 55-year-old male patient came with complaints of rapidly progressive dementia and altered sensorium over past 3 months. **(A–F)** MRI shows asymmetrical cortical FLAIR hyperintensity with diffusion restriction is in bilateral fronto-parietal and occipital cortices (white arrows) with relative sparing of peri-Rolandic region.

10

Neurotrauma

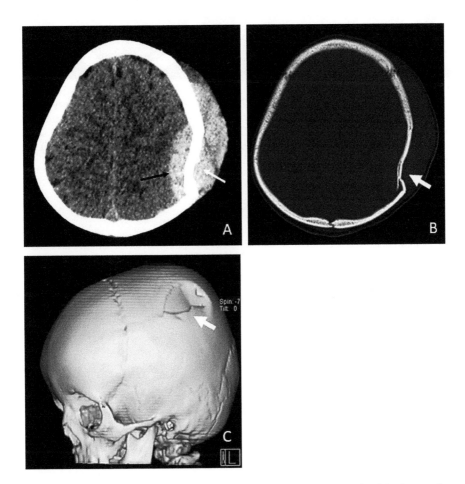

Figure 10.1 Extradural hematoma (EDH) with depressed fracture: **(A)** Axial NCCT brain of a
34-year-old female who suffered a road traffic accident (RTA), shows lentiform shaped extradural
(black arrow) and subgaleal hematoma (white arrow) in left fronto-parietal region (white arrow).
(B) Axial bone window and **(C)** VRT images show depressed fracture in left parietal bone (thick white
arrow). EDH is usually associated with adjacent bone fracture in three-fourth of the cases. EDH does
not cross the suture line as it is subperiosteal in nature which helps to differentiate it from subdural
hemorrhage.

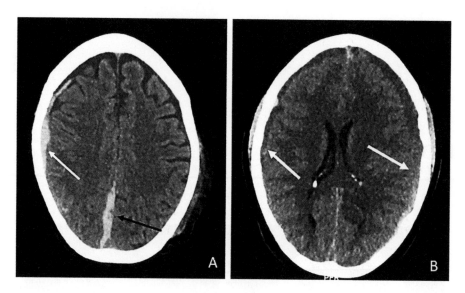

Figure 10.2 Subdural hematoma (SDH): **(A)** Axial NCCT head of a patient with history of road traffic accident shows crescentshaped hemorrhage, representing acute SDH in right frontoparietal convexity (white arrow) and posterior falx (black arrow). **(B)** Second image (of a different patient) shows subacute on chronic subdural hematoma in both cerebral convexities (thick white arrow). SDH may cross sutures, unlike EDH.

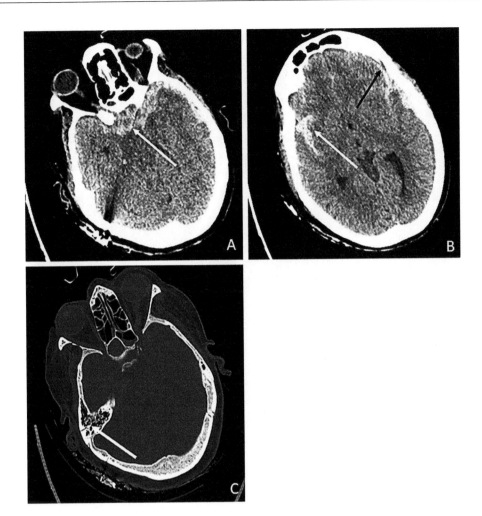

Figure 10.3 Traumatic subarachnoid hemorrhage (SAH): **(A, B)** Axial NCCT images of brain of a 63-year-old female who presented with loss of consciousness (LOC), vomiting and, ear bleed after RTA showing subarachnoid hemorrhage (thin white arrow) in basal cisterns and both Sylvian fissures and thin SDH (black arrow) along left temporal convexity. **(C)** Axial NCCT bone window shows linear fracture in mastoid part of right temporal bone (thick white arrow). Trauma is the most common cause of the SAH followed by aneurysmal rupture.

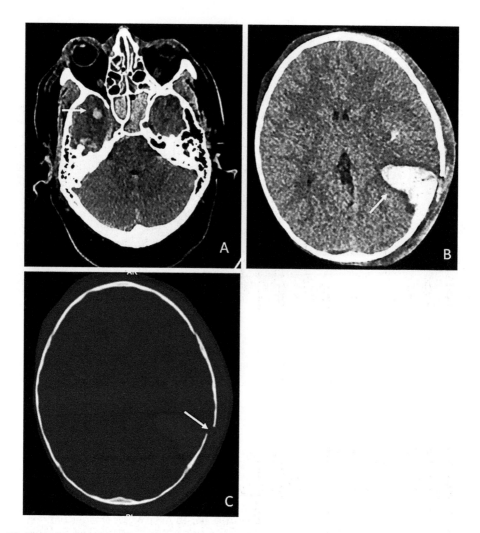

Figure 10.4 Hemorrhagic contusion: **(A, B)** Axial NCCT of head of a 22-year-old young male with road traffic accident (RTA) shows hemorrhagic contusions in left parietal lobe, left putamen, and right anterior temporal lobe (white arrows). Note the other associated injuries such as sphenoid hemosinus, right preseptal, and left temporo-parietal subgaleal soft tissue swelling. **(C)** Linear minimally displaced fracture in left parietal bone is seen in bone window images (white arrow).

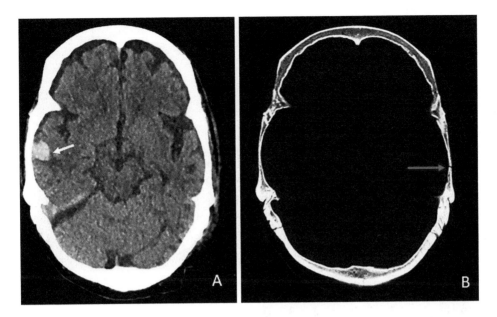

Figure 10.5 Coup–contrecoup injury: A 60-year-old male with history of RTA, **(A)** Axial NCCT images of both brain and bone window **(B)** show linear fracture in left temporal lobe (red arrow) indicating the point of impact. Hemorrhagic contusions are seen in the right temporal lobe (white arrow), which is located opposite to the site of primary impact. These injuries are commonly associated with differential acceleration of the brain structures with respect to the calvarium after the initial impact.

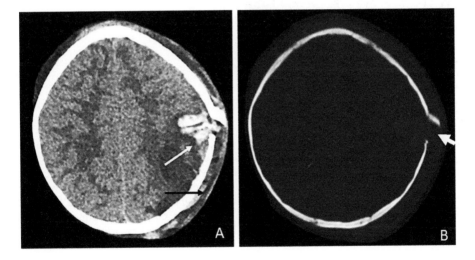

Figure 10.6 Elevated fracture with contusion: **(A, B)** Axial NCCT images of the brain and bone window show elevated fracture (thick white arrow) with adjacent hemorrhagic contusions (thin white arrow) in left posterior frontal lobe with adjacent non-hemorrhagic contusions and edema. Note is also made of subgaleal soft tissue swelling (black arrow).

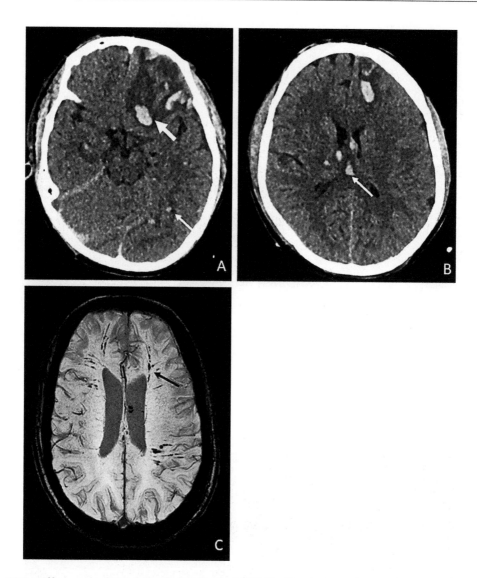

Figure 10.7 Diffuse axonal injury (DAI): **(A, B)** Axial NCCT of brain shows hemorrhagic contusions in left basifrontal lobe (thick white arrow) at the site of primary impact. Multiple punctate hemorrhagic contusions in both temporal, left occipital and in the body and splenium of the corpus callosum (thin white arrow). **(C)** Axial SWI image showed multiple linear and punctate foci of blooming in gray-white matter junction of both frontal and parietal lobe (black arrow) and near body of the corpus callosum. Punctate hemorrhagic contusions in gray-white matter junction, corpus callosum, and brainstem are characteristic of diffuse axonal injury. Patients with DAI usually have a poorer outcome.

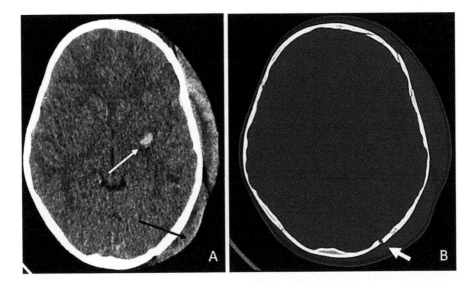

Figure 10.8 Diffuse axonal injury with fracture: **(A, B)** Axial NCCT of brain and bone window of a 34-year-old female presented with RTA and poor GCS shows hemorrhagic contusion in left basal ganglia (thin white arrow) with subgaleal contusion in fronto-temporo-parietal scalp (thin black arrow). Linear minimally displaced fracture on the left side of the occipital bone (thick white arrow). Deep gray nuclei contusions can occur in absence of superficial cortical contusions and carries poor prognosis.

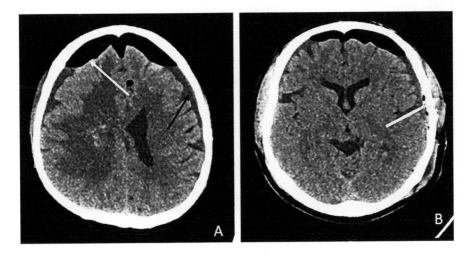

Figure 10.9 Pneumocephalus: **(A, B)** Axial NCCT of head of a 56-year-old male presented with RTA shows areas of air densities (thin white arrow) in both anterior frontal convexities and falx suggestive of pneumocephalus (Mount Fuji sign). Subdural collection (thin black arrow) in both fronto-temporal convexities. Note is also made of subgaleal soft tissue swelling in both temporal region (thick white arrow).

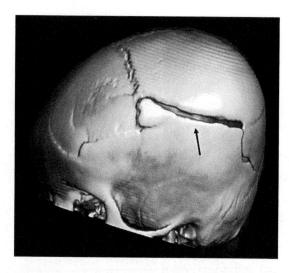

Figure 10.10 Linear fracture: 3D volume-rendered image of a 26-year-old female presented with RTA shows linear undisplaced fracture (black arrow) in left parietal bone extending from coronal suture to lambdoid suture. Linear fractures are the commonest type of skull fractures. Fractures can indicate severity of trauma.

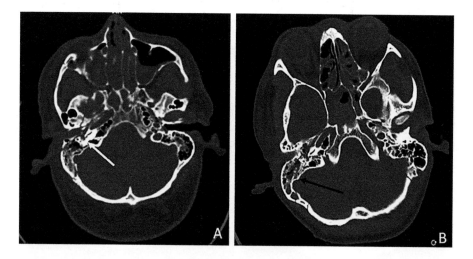

Figure 10.11 Temporal bone fracture: (A, B) Axial NCCT images of a 38-year-old female presented with RTA skull at the level of temporal bone show linear undisplaced fracture (thin white arrow) extending from right occipital bone to squamous part of the right temporal bone with involvement of mastoid part of right temporal bone. Note is made of collection in right middle ear and mastoid air cells (black arrow) with hemosinus. Mastoid fractures are commonly associated with bleeding from the ear.

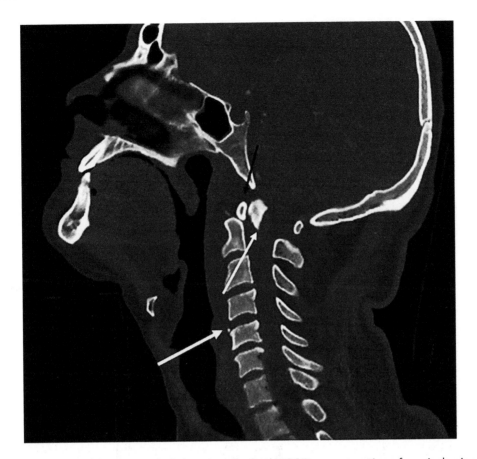

Figure 10.12 Odontoid fracture with dislocation: Sagittal NCCT reconstruction of cervical spine of a 54-year-old male presented with trauma shows fracture with posterior dislocation of dens (thin white arrow) causing bony spinal canal narrowing and possible spinal cord compression. Posterior dislocation (black arrow) of anterior arch of atlas is also seen. Note is also made of extension tear drop fracture at upper end plate of C5 vertebral body (thick white arrow).

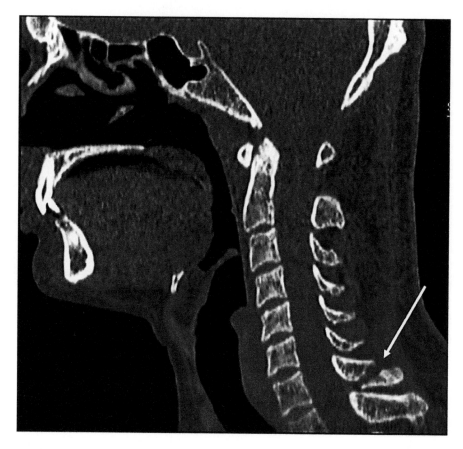

Figure 10.13 Clay-shoveler's fracture: Sagittal NCCT reconstruction of cervical spine of a 38-year-old male presented with RTA shows linear partially displaced fracture (white arrow) of C7 spinous process. Note is made of intact normal cervical lordotic curvature and intact vertebral bodies. This type of fracture occurs due to hyperextension injury and is considered as a stable fracture.

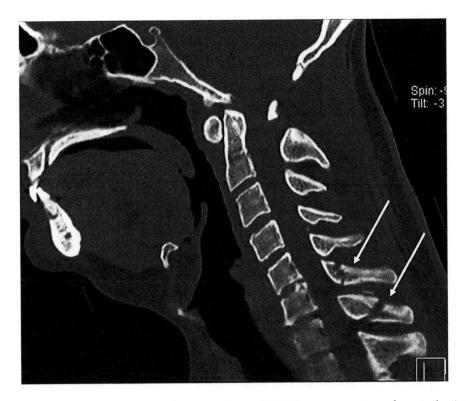

Figure 10.14 Multiple spinous process fractures: Sagittal NCCT reconstruction of cervical spine of a 50-year-old male presented with road traffic accident shows linear partially displaced fractures (thin white arrow) involving spinous processes of C6 & C7 vertebra. Note is made of loss of normal cervical lordosis with intact vertebral bodies. Mechanism of this injury is hyperflexion of neck.

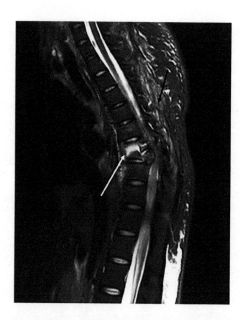

Figure 10.15 Burst fracture: Sagittal T2-w MRI of a 23-year-old female presented with RTA shows burst fracture (white arrow) of D8 vertebral body with retropulsion of fractured segment causing spinal canal stenosis. Altered signal intensity is seen within the spinal cord, above and below the level of fractured segment. Note is also made of interspinous ligamentous edema (black arrow). This type of fracture occurs due to extensive shearing force to spine.

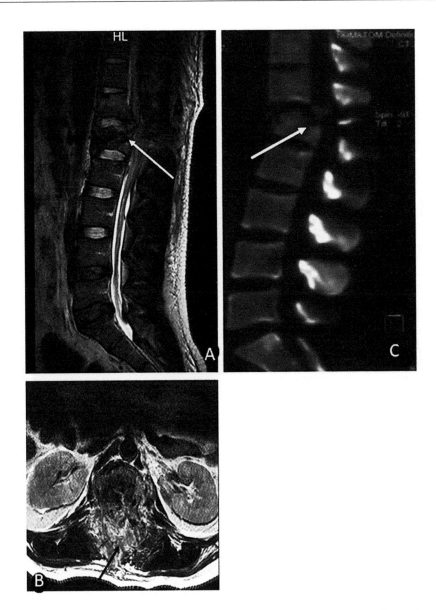

Figure 10.16 Burst fracture with posterior ligamentous complex (PLC) injury: **(A)** Sagittal and **(B)** axial T2 MRI of lumbar spine of a 33-year-old female presented with RTA shows L1 burst fracture (thin white arrow) with retropulsion of fractured segment causing spinal cord compression. Note is made of involvement of posterior ligamentous complex (PLC) as hyperintensity and edema (thin black arrow). **(C)** Sagittal NCCT image of the same patient shows L1 burst fracture (thick white arrow) with retropulsion of the fractured segment. Note is also made of fracture of posterior spinous process. Transversely oriented fractures involving Denis 3 columns are known as chance fractures.

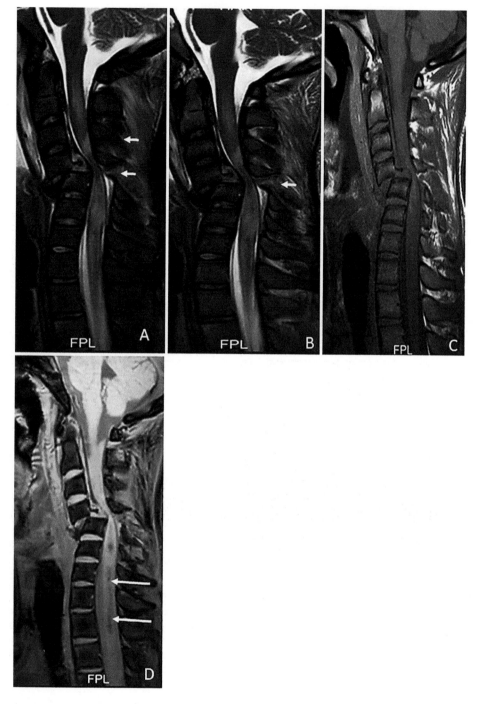

Figure 10.17 Hemorrhagic contusion of the cord in severe cervical spine trauma: A 22-year-old male presented with road traffic accident. **(A)** Sagittal T2 and **(B)** STIR images show anterolisthesis of C4 over C5 vertebra with spinal canal stenosis and hyperintensity within the spinal cord. Posterior ligamentous complex (PLC) injury is seen as rupture of ligamentum flavum and hyperintensity within interspinous and supraspinous ligaments (small white arrows). **(C)** Sagittal T1 image shows no hyperintensity within the spinal cord. **(D)** Sagittal MERGE image shows focal and linear blooming within the spinal cord at and below the level of injury suggestive of hemorrhagic contusions (long white arrow). Hemorrhagic contusions within the cord signify poor prognosis.

11

Degenerative brain and spine diseases

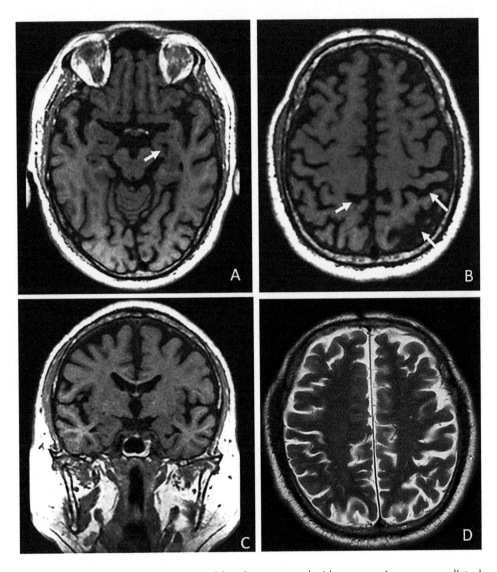

Figure 11.1 Alzheimer's disease: A 63-year-old male presented with progressive memory disturbances. **(A, B)** Axial, **(C)** coronal T1-w, and **(D)** axial T2-w images show asymmetrical atrophy of the cerebral parenchyma predominantly involving temporal and parietal lobes. These are evident by asymmetric prominence of sulcal spaces in the temporal and parietal lobes (white arrows).

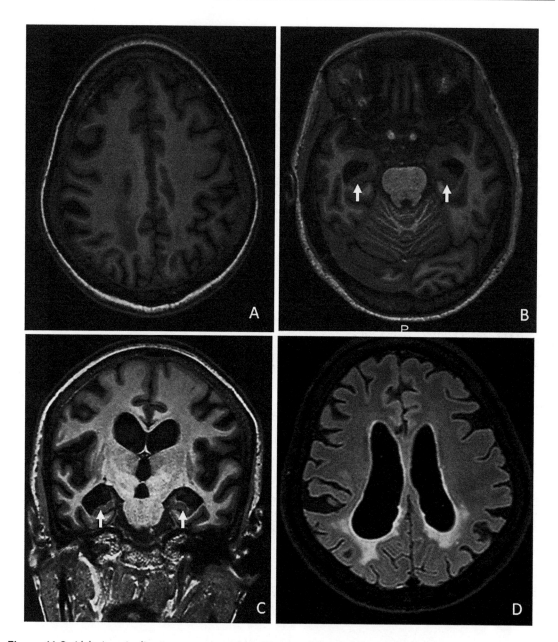

Figure 11.2 Alzheimer's disease – continued: A 65-year-old male presented with visual agnosia and memory disturbances for the past 2 years. **(A, B)** Axial, **(C)** coronal T1-w, and **(D)** axial FLAIR images show selective atrophy of the medial temporal lobes and parietal lobes. Hippocampal volume loss (white arrows) is seen with dilatation of temporal horns of both lateral ventricles, and parietal volume loss is evidenced by asymmetric dilatation of atrium and posterior body of both lateral ventricles. Periventricular white matter signal changes are also evident in the parietal white matter.

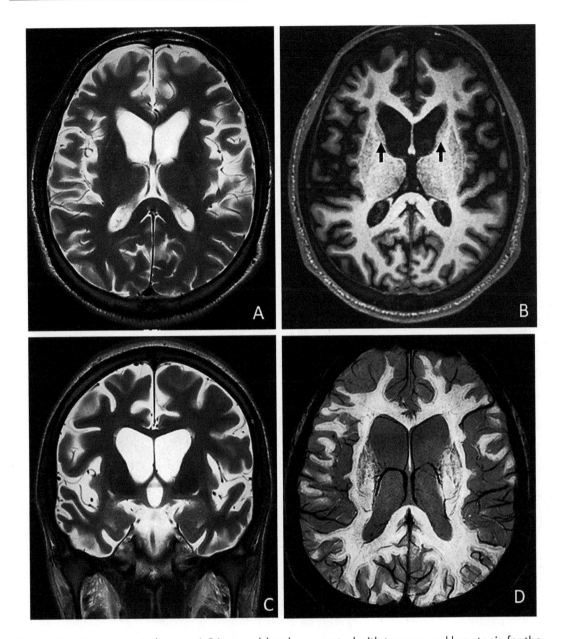

Figure 11.3 Huntington's disease: A 34-year-old male presented with tremors and hypotonia for the last 16 years. **(A)** Axial T2, **(B)** T1, and **(C)** coronal T2-w images show atrophy of both caudate nuclei and putamen without obvious signal abnormality (black arrows). Bilateral symmetric atrophy of both cerebral parenchyma is seen, predominantly affecting both frontal and anterior temporal lobes. **(D)** SWI image shows a few blooming foci in the region of both caudate and putamina.

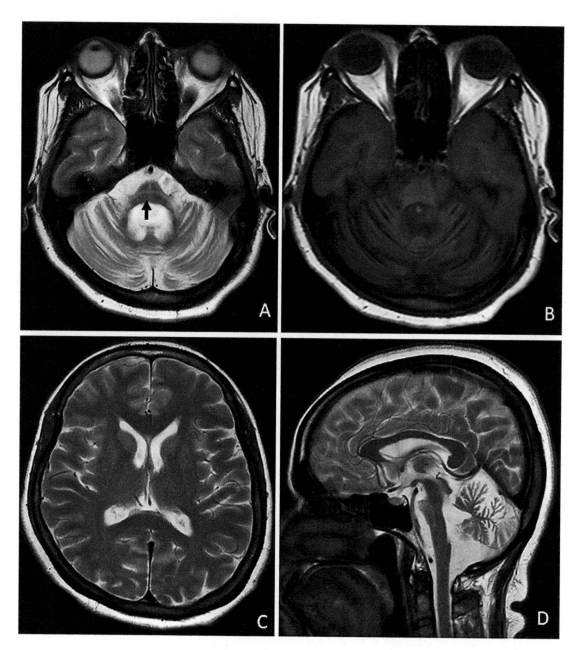

Figure 11.4 Multiple system atrophy-C (MSA-C): A 50-year-old female presented with progressive cerebellar ataxia since 4 years. **(A)** Axial T2 and **(B)** T1-w images at the level of brainstem show diffuse cerebellar, middle cerebellar peduncle, and brainstem atrophy with hyperintensity along pontocerebellar tracts (hot-cross bun sign) (black arrow). **(C)** Axial T2-w image at the level of basal ganglia is unremarkable. **(D)** Sagittal T2-w image shows brainstem and vermian atrophy.

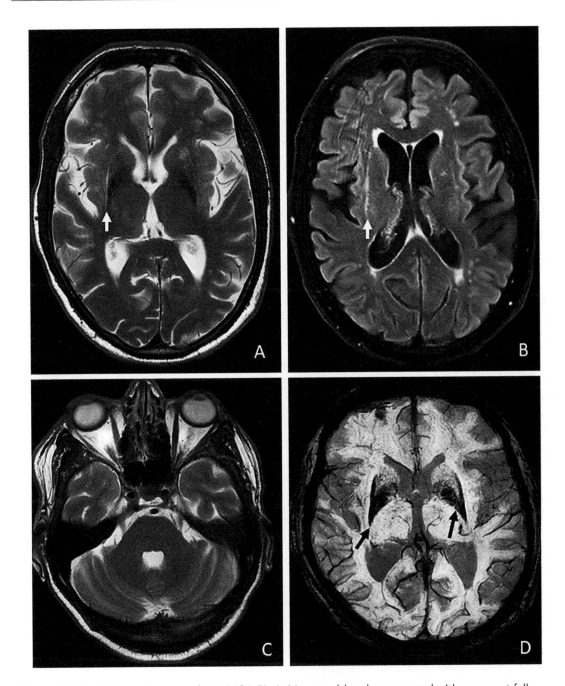

Figure 11.5 Multiple system atrophy-P (MSA-P): A 66-year-old male presented with recurrent falls. (A) Axial T2 and (B) FLAIR images show symmetric volume loss in both putamina with hyperintensity along lateral aspect (bright putamina sign) (white arrows). (C) Axial T2-w image at the level of brainstem shows no significant abnormality. (D) SWI image shows blooming in the mid and posterior aspect of both lentiform nuclei (black arrows).

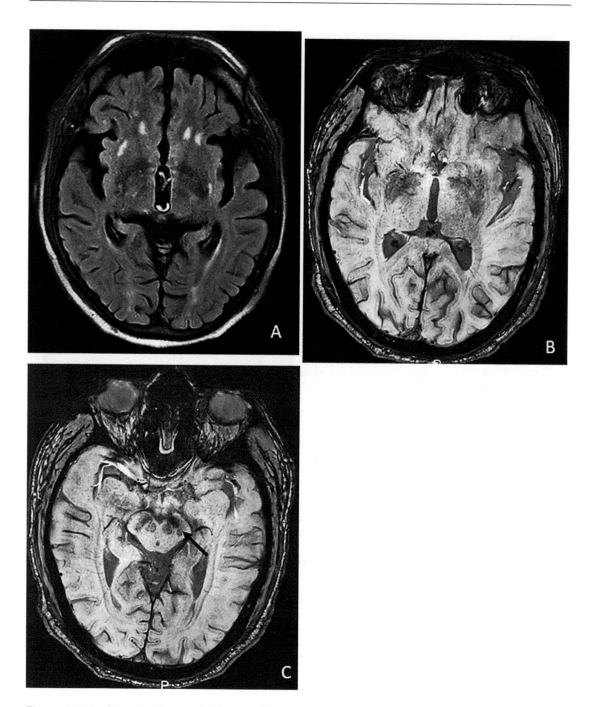

Figure 11.6 Parkinson's disease: A 56-year-old male presented with slowness of gait, difficulty in walking, and rigidity in all four limbs. (A, B) Axial FLAIR image shows hypointensity in both globus pallidus due to abnormal mineral deposition. Focal bright areas in both basifrontal lobes and anterior aspect of right external capsule may represent coexisting. Note is made of small vessel ischemic changes. (C) Axial SWI image shows loss of swallow tail sign (black arrow) in midbrain due to loss of nigrosome and abnormal mineral deposition in both globus pallidus.

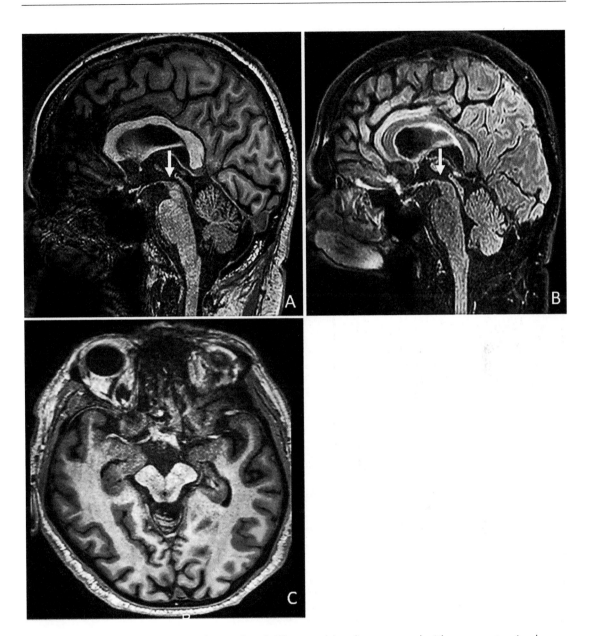

Figure 11.7 Progressive supranuclear palsy: A 56-year-old male presented with recurrent episodes of falls and tremors. (A) Sagittal FLAIR and (B) T1-w images show flattening with mild concavity in superior surface of midbrain (white arrow). (C) Axial T1-w image shows concave appearing lateral margin of brainstem.

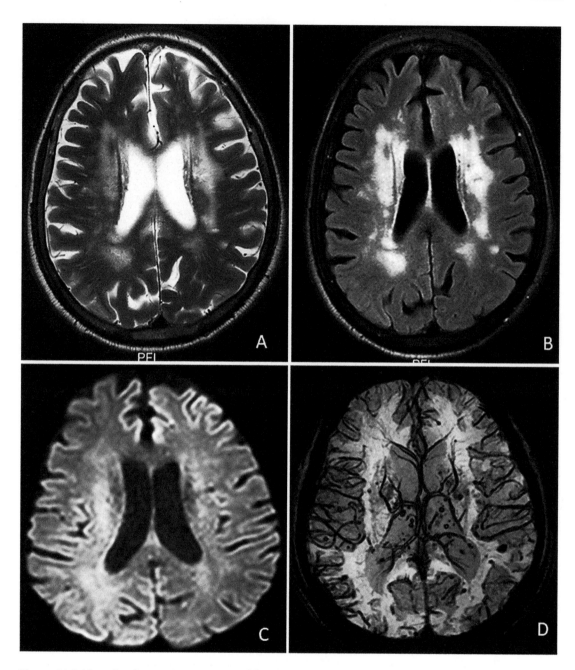

Figure 11.8 Vascular dementia: A 64-year-old male, known hypertensive, presented with recurrent neurologic deficits and memory loss. **(A)** Axial T2 and **(B)** FLAIR images show multiple confluent and discrete hyperintensities in both frontal and parietal lobe white matter with mid diffuse cerebral atrophy. **(C)** Axial DWI image shows no acute infarcts and **(D)** SWI image shows multiple foci of microhemorrhages in cortex and basal ganglia.

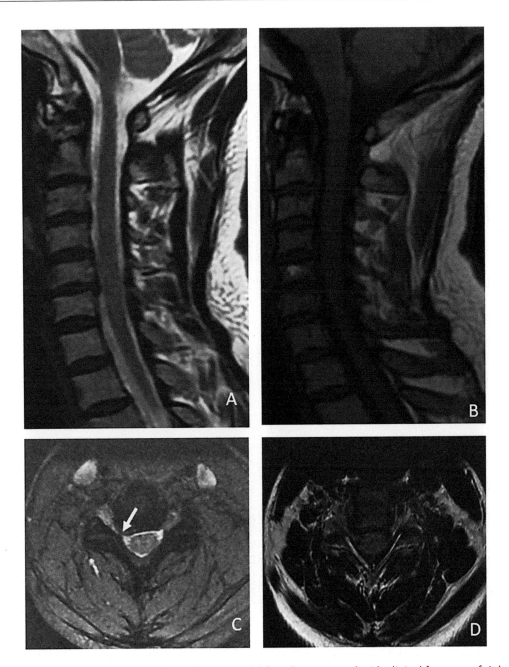

Figure 11.9 Cervical spine disc bulge: A 46-year-old female presented with clinical features of right C5-C6 radiculopathy. **(A)** Sagittal T2 and **(B)** T1-w images show reduced disc height at C5-C6 level with indentation of thecal sac without spinal canal narrowing. **(C)** Axial MERGE and **(D)** T2-w images show right neural foraminal narrowing with indentation of right C6 exiting nerve root (white arrow). Note is made of desiccative changes (disc dehydration) in all cervical intervertebral discs.

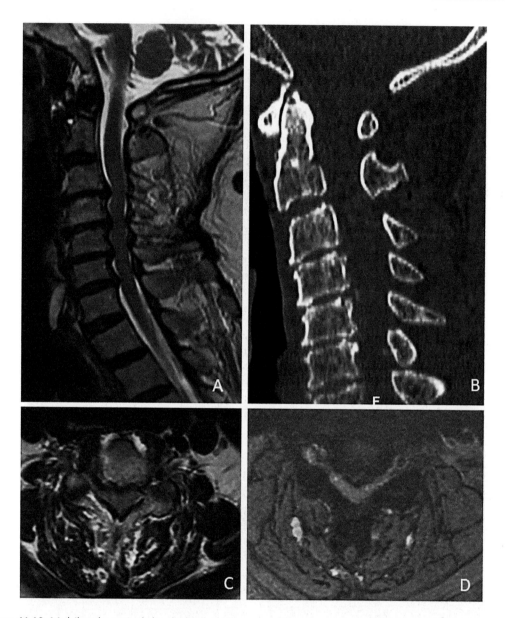

Figure 11.10 Multilevel cervical disc bulge: A 62-year-old female presented with neck pain and weakness involving both upper limbs. **(A)** Sagittal T2-w image shows multilevel disc bulge at C3-C4 to C6-C7 levels with spinal canal stenosis and cord compression. **(B)** Axial T2 and **(C)** MERGE images show spinal canal compromise and cord compression. **(D)** Sagittal CT reconstruction of the cervical spine shows disco-osteophyte complex with degenerative changes in spine. Note the ligamentum hypertrophy at lower cervical levels.

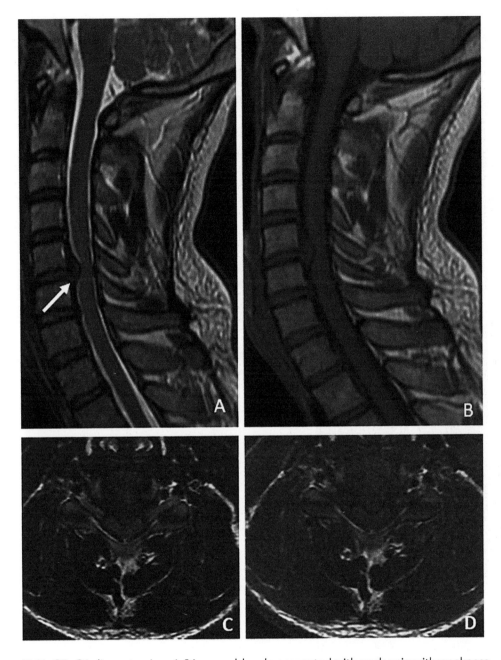

Figure 11.11 C5–C6 disc extrusion: A 36-year-old male presented with neck pain with weakness involving both upper limbs. **(A)** Sagittal T2 and **(B)** T1-w images show disc extrusion at C5–C6 level with spinal cord compression (white arrow). **(C)** Axial T2 and **(D)** T1-w images at the same level show significant spinal canal stenosis and cord compression.

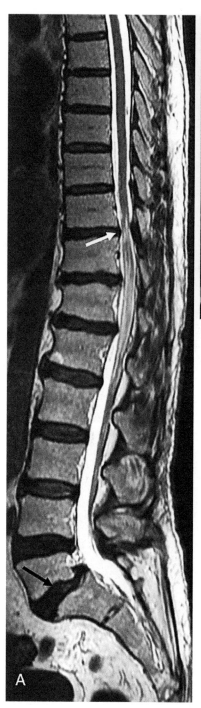

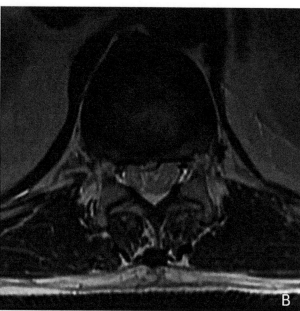

Figure 11.12 Dorsal disc herniation: A 63-year-old male presented with both lower limb weakness for the past 2 years. **(A)** Sagittal and **(B)** axial T2-w images show disc bulges at D10-D11 and D11-D12 with spinal canal compromise and signal change in the spinal cord (white arrow). Note is made of ligamentum flavum hypertrophy at D10-D11 level and grade 1 anterolisthesis L5 over S1 vertebra (black arrow).

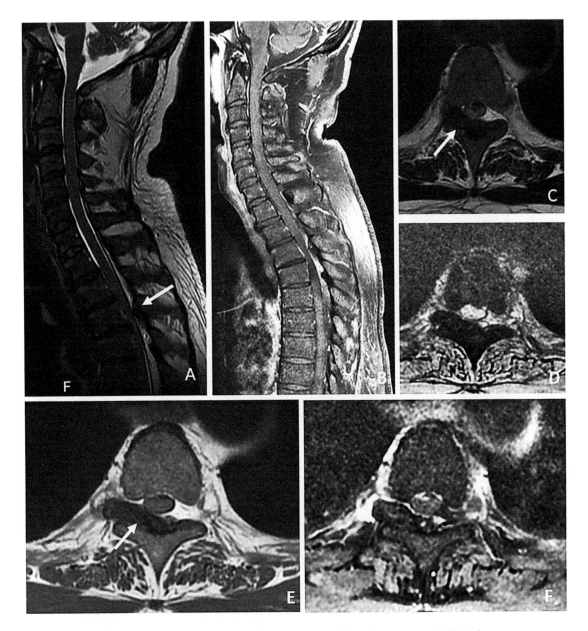

Figure 11.13 Ligamentum flavum hypertrophy: A 46-year-old male presented with right upper and lower limb weakness since 4 months. **(A)** Sagittal T2 and **(B)** T1-w post-contrast images show ligamentum flavum hypertrophy at right D3-D4 level, causing neural foraminal narrowing and cord compression (white arrows). No enhancement is seen after contrast administration. **(C)** Axial T2 and **(D)** MERGE images show spinal canal compromise and cord compression. **(E)** Axial T1 pre- and **(F)** post-contrast images show no significant enhancement. Note is made of multilevel disc bulges at cervical level.

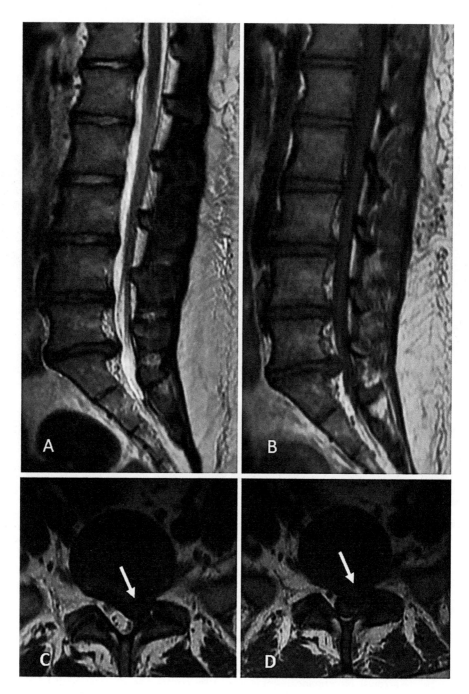

Figure 11.14 Lumbar disc protrusion: A 25-year-old male presented with increase in pain and weakness in left lower limb since 4 months. **(A)** Sagittal T2 and **(B)** T1-w images show disc protrusion at L5-S1 level with spinal canal stenosis. **(C)** Axial T2 and **(D)** T1-w images show disc protrusion with left lateral recess and spinal canal stenosis and entrapment of left L5 exiting and S1 traversing nerve roots (white arrows).

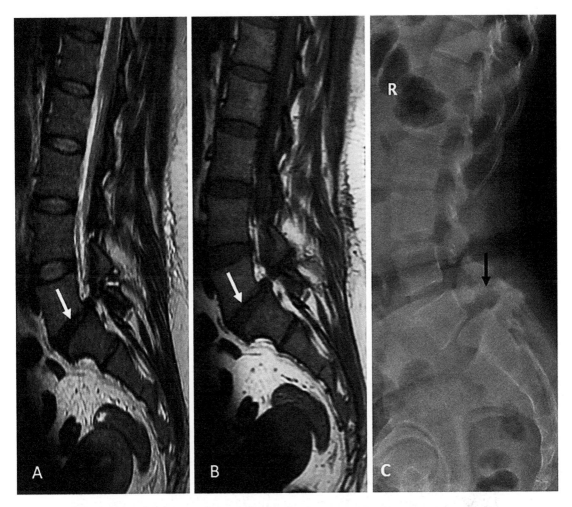

Figure 11.15 Spondylolisthesis: A 42-year-old male presented with low back pain for the past 1 year. **(A)** Sagittal T2 and **(B)** T1-w images show grade 1 spondylolisthesis of L5 over S1 vertebra (white arrows), with bony defect in both pars interarticularis of L5. Disc bulge is seen at the same level with spinal canal stenosis. **(C)** Lumbar spine lateral view (weight-bearing) shows grade 2 anterolisthesis with bilateral pars interarticularis defects at the same level (black arrow).

Index